Pain: The Universal Feeling

OrangeBooks Publication

1st Floor, Rajhans Arcade, Mall Road, Kohka, Bhilai, Chhattisgarh 490020

Website: **www.orangebooks.in**

First Edition, 2025

ISBN: 978-93-6554-758-0

Price: Rs. 350.00

Printed in India

PAIN

The Universal Feeling

DR. KALPANA K

OrangeBooks Publication
www.orangebooks.in

Introduction

Pain: The Universal Feeling

By Dr. Kalpana K

FIPP (USA), FIAPM, Gold Medalist in FIAPM

Pain is a language every human understands—a universal feeling that transcends age, culture, and geography. Yet, for something so deeply personal and common, it remains shrouded in myths, misconceptions, and stigma.

As a pain specialist with over 14 years of experience, I have seen pain in its many forms: the sharp, sudden sting of acute discomfort, the relentless ache of chronic suffering, and the invisible pain that society often overlooks. Through my journey, supported by credentials like FIPP (USA) and FIAPM (Gold Medalist), I have committed myself to understanding and addressing pain in its entirety.

In my practice and as a Governing Council member of the Indian Society for Study of Pain's Karnataka State Chapter, I have come to realize that pain is more than a physical sensation—it is a story shaped by biology, emotions, and social perceptions. The goal of this book is to help you unravel that story and rewrite it on your terms.

This book, Pain: The Universal Feeling, is a culmination of years spent working on the frontlines of medicine. It aims to empower you with insights into the nature of pain, its origins, and its impact on your life. From the latest breakthroughs in science to time-tested holistic approaches, we'll explore practical ways to navigate and overcome pain.

But this is also a call to rethink how we, as individuals and a society, view pain. It's time to shift the narrative from mere survival to healing and thriving. Pain may be universal, but it doesn't have to define us.

Whether you are a patient, a caregiver, or someone seeking to understand this complex experience better, this book is for you. Together, we'll challenge the misconceptions, demystify the science, and unlock the possibility of a life beyond pain.

Let's embark on this journey together to reclaim hope, resilience, and the promise of a pain-free tomorrow

Table Of Contents

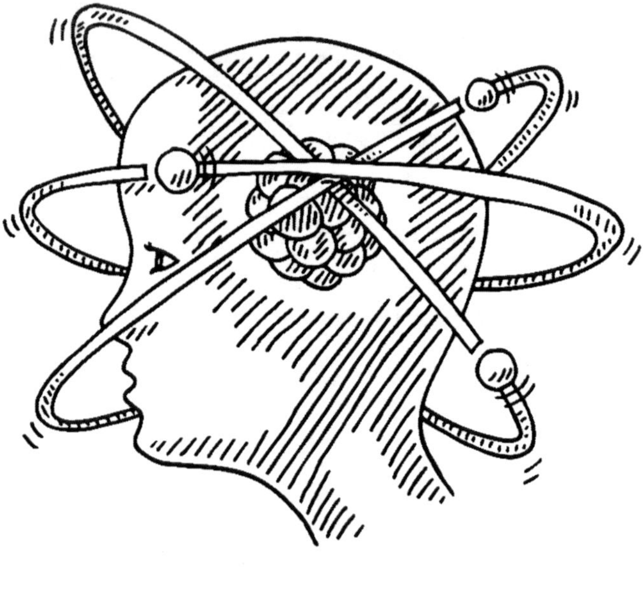

Chapter - 1
Redefining Pain

1.1 Pain as a Signal, Not a Symptom

As a pain specialist, I've come to understand pain as much more than just discomfort. It's a signal—a message your body is trying to send you. In my years of practice, I've seen countless patients who initially wanted nothing more than to "make the pain stop." However, it's important to understand that pain is not an enemy. It's your body's way of asking for attention, and ignoring it can often make things worse.

Pain functions similarly to a smoke alarm. If your house catches fire, the alarm is there to alert you so you can act quickly. Now imagine disabling that alarm without addressing the fire. The flames will only spread. This is exactly what happens when we silence pain with quick fixes like painkillers, painkillers without understanding the root cause.

The Protective Role of Pain

Pain has saved lives. I've seen patients who came to me with persistent, unexplained pain only to discover underlying conditions that needed urgent attention. For example, one patient of mine—a young professional in her 30s—had been experiencing constant shoulder pain.

She thought it was due to her poor posture at work. However, after some deeper investigation, we discovered she was in the early stages of rheumatoid arthritis. Her pain wasn't just an inconvenience; it was her body's way of signaling a deeper problem.

Pain plays three critical roles in our lives:

1. **Warning Us of Danger**: Like the sharp jolt you feel when you touch a hot stove, pain prevents us from causing further harm to ourselves.

2. **Guiding Recovery**: That tender feeling in an injured area reminds you to protect it, giving your body the time it needs to heal.

3. **Uncovering Hidden Issues**: Chronic pain can be the first sign of something serious—nerve damage, inflammation, or even an autoimmune disorder.

Misunderstanding Pain

Too often, I meet patients who see pain as an adversary. They're frustrated and desperate to silence it. And while I completely understand—pain can be exhausting and overwhelming—ignoring what it's trying to tell you is like covering your ears when someone's shouting, "Look out!"

Take headaches, for example. They're one of the most common complaints I hear. Many people simply take a pill and move on. But headaches can tell us so much: Are you dehydrated? Are you under constant stress? Is there an issue with your vision? The pain itself isn't the problem—it's a clue.

Learning to Listen

As a doctor, I've learned to interpret pain in its own unique language. Sharp, stabbing pain often points to an injury. Dull, aching pain can mean inflammation. Pain that radiates might indicate a nerve issue. Widespread pain may even be a sign of something systemic, like fibromyalgia.

When you understand pain as a signal, it transforms the way you approach it. Instead of asking, *"How do I stop this pain?"* ask, *"What is my body trying to tell me?"*

1.2 Beyond Physical: Pain and the Mind-Body Nexus

The mind deeply intertwines with pain, making it more than just a physical sensation. Over the years, I have seen this connection play out in ways that scicncc is only beginning to understand fully. The pain you feel in your body is inseparable from the thoughts, emotions, and experiences that shape your reality. It is not "all in your head," but it is also not just in your body—it is both.

The Mind's Role in Pain

Pain begins as a signal in the body, but it is the brain that decides how to interpret it. For instance, when you stub your toe, nerve endings send signals to your brain saying, *"Something's wrong!"* But the brain doesn't just process that information mechanically. It asks additional questions: *How bad is this? Have I experienced this before? Am I safe?*

This process explains why two people with the same injury can experience vastly different levels of pain. One may describe it as a mild discomfort, while the other feels it as unbearable agony. Their brains interpret the signal differently based on factors like stress, past trauma, and even mood.

The Feedback Loop Between Pain and Emotion

Pain and emotions are part of a feedback loop that can either help or harm. Chronic pain, for example, can lead to feelings of frustration, anxiety, and even depression. These emotions, in turn, amplify the sensation of pain, creating a vicious cycle.

Here's why: emotions like fear or stress heighten the brain's sensitivity to pain signals. When you're anxious, your body releases stress hormones such as cortisol, which can make your nerves more reactive. This heightened sensitivity means the same pain signal feels much worse than it would if you were calm and relaxed.

Conversely, positive emotions have the opposite effect. Joy, laughter, and a sense of purpose can reduce pain by releasing endorphins, your body's natural painkillers. This isn't wishful thinking—it's biology.

Chronic Pain and the Mind-Body Disconnect

In chronic pain conditions, the mind-body connection becomes even more complex. Chronic pain often persists long after the original injury has healed, suggesting that the pain signals are no longer just about tissue damage. Instead, the brain and nervous system have become stuck in a pattern of heightened alertness, constantly perceiving danger where none exists.

We refer to this phenomenon as central sensitization.It's as if the brain has turned up the volume on pain signals, making even light touches feel unbearable. Breaking this cycle requires addressing not just the physical causes of pain but also the psychological ones.

The Power of Awareness

One of the most transformative approaches I have seen is teaching patients to become aware of their mind-body connection. This is not about ignoring physical pain or suggesting that it's "just mental." Instead, it's about recognizing that our thoughts, emotions, and physical sensations are all part of the same system.

For instance, studies have shown that mindfulness helps patients observe their pain without passing judgment, thereby reducing chronic pain. When you stop fighting pain and start listening to it, something remarkable happens: the pain often loses its grip.

Moving Toward Holistic Healing

The mind-body connection is why holistic approaches to pain management—those that address both physical and emotional well-being—are so effective. Practices like meditation, cognitive-behavioral therapy, and even journaling about your pain can help rewire the brain to perceive it differently. At the same time, it's essential to combine these practices with medical interventions. Addressing the physical causes of pain without considering the emotional toll is incomplete, just as focusing solely on the mind ignores the reality of bodily suffering.

Pain is never just physical or just mental—it is both. Understanding this nexus allows us to treat pain more effectively, not by compartmentalizing it but by addressing it as the multifaceted experience it truly is. This approach doesn't just reduce pain; it empowers you to take control of your healing journey.

1.3 Chronic vs. Episodic Pain: The Gray Area

As a pain specialist, one of the most common questions I encounter is, *"Why doesn't my pain go away?"* To answer this, we must understand the distinction between chronic and episodic pain—and the complex space in between, which I often refer to as *the gray area.*

Pain is not a universal experience. Some pain is fleeting, while other types linger, resist treatment, and shape lives in ways we often underestimate. By defining these forms of pain and exploring their overlap, I hope to shed light on what you may be experiencing and why.

What is Episodic Pain?

Episodic pain is a type of pain that fluctuates and is often triggered by specific events or conditions. A classic example is a headache. You might have a headache after staring at a screen for too long or skipping a meal. The pain usually subsides with rest, hydration, or over-the-counter medication.

This type of pain serves as a signal—your body's way of saying, *"Something needs attention."* Addressing the trigger resolves the pain and returns life to normal.

Episodic pain can feel intense in the moment, but it is generally short-lived. It acts as a messenger, warning you of potential harm or imbalance.

Understanding Chronic Pain

On the other hand, chronic pain presents a unique challenge. Defined as pain lasting longer than the three months, it often persists long after the original injury or illness has healed. For patients living with chronic pain, the sensation becomes a constant companion—a relentless reminder of discomfort and limitation.

Unlike episodic pain, chronic pain is not merely a warning signal. In many cases, it serves no protective purpose. Instead, it reflects changes in the nervous system, where the pain pathways become overactive and hypersensitive.

Chronic pain can stem from a variety of conditions:

- **Arthritis:** Pain from joint inflammation that never fully subsides.
- **Neuropathy:** Nerve pain often associated with diabetes or injury.
- **Fibromyalgia:** Widespread pain with no clear physical cause.

Living with chronic pain is not just a physical challenge; it's an emotional and psychological one as well. Patients often face feelings of isolation, frustration, and even despair.

The Gray Area: When Pain is Neither Fully Chronic Nor Episodic

Pain doesn't always fit neatly into the categories of chronic or episodic. Many of my patients find themselves in this gray area, where pain seems to shift unpredictably.

Take, for instance, someone with recurring migraines. The pain is episodic, but the frequency and severity can feel chronic. Similarly, conditions such as irritable bowel syndrome (IBS) or lower back pain frequently blur the boundaries, alternating between periods of relief and flare-ups.

This gray area is especially challenging because it defies straightforward treatment. Patients often ask, *"Is this going to go away, or will it stay with me forever?"* The answer is rarely simple.

Why Does Pain Persist?

Understanding why pain becomes chronic or fluctuates between chronic and episodic requires looking beyond the initial cause. Factors that contribute to persistent pain include:

- **Central Sensitization:** The nervous system becomes overly sensitive, amplifying pain signals.
- **Inflammation:** Chronic low-grade inflammation can sustain pain over time.
- **Lifestyle Factors:** Poor sleep, stress, and sedentary habits can exacerbate pain.

- **Psychological Triggers:** Anxiety, depression, and past trauma often heighten pain perception.

This interplay of physical, psychological, and lifestyle factors creates a complex web that sustains pain, making it resistant to traditional treatments.

Moving from Categorization to Care

While labels like "chronic" and "episodic" are helpful for diagnosis, they don't tell the full story of your pain. The goal is not just to categorize pain but to understand its unique characteristics and underlying causes.

In my practice, I focus on a comprehensive approach that includes:

1. **Identifying Triggers:** Tracking when and why pain occurs.
2. **Customizing Treatment:** Combining medical interventions, physical therapy, and lifestyle changes.
3. **Addressing Mental Health:** Incorporating counseling or mindfulness techniques to reduce the emotional toll of pain.
4. **Empowering Patients:** Educating patients to take an active role in their own recovery.

Living Beyond Pain

Whether your pain is chronic, episodic, or somewhere in between, it does not define you. It is a part of your story, but not the whole narrative. By understanding the nuances of pain and addressing it with care and compassion, we can find ways to improve your quality of life—even if the pain itself doesn't entirely go away.

In this gray area, hope lies in persistence, patience, and the belief that progress, no matter how small, is always possible.

1.4 The Role of Genetics in Pain Perception

When we talk about pain, most of us think of it in terms of injury or illness—a stubbed toe, a pulled muscle, a back strain. However, there's a hidden layer to pain perception that many don't consider: our genetic makeup. Genetics plays a crucial role in how we experience pain, influencing everything from the intensity of pain we feel to our response to pain treatments.

Why Genetics Matters in Pain

Pain perception is not just about physical injury. It's a complex process that involves the nervous system, brain, and even genetic predispositions. While some people are genetically predisposed to certain diseases, others may be more sensitive to pain.

Our genes can influence

1. **Pain Threshold:** The level of stimulus required for someone to perceive pain.
2. **Pain Tolerance:** The ability to endure pain once it's felt.
3. **Chronic Pain Development:** Some people's genetic makeup increases their risk of developing chronic

pain conditions, even after the initial injury has healed.

Essentially, pain is not a purely external experience; it's shaped by internal factors—many of which are encoded in our DNA.

Genetic Variations and Pain Sensitivity

Scientific research has identified several genetic variations that can affect pain sensitivity. These variations can impact how our bodies process pain signals and the strength of those signals.

- **Ion Channels:** These are proteins in our cells that control the flow of ions and help transmit pain signals. Variations in genes that code for ion channels, like the **SCN9A gene**, have been linked to increased pain sensitivity or reduced pain perception.
- **Endorphin Receptors:** Endorphins are the body's natural painkillers, and some genetic variations can make people more or less responsive to these pain-relieving substances. Those with certain genetic profiles may experience less relief from painkillers, even if their bodies produce enough endorphins.
- **Inflammation Response:** Genes involved in inflammation (like the **C-reactive protein gene**) can also play a role in pain sensitivity. People with specific genetic variations may experience heightened pain in response to inflammation, which is common in conditions like arthritis.

The Genetic Basis of Chronic Pain

One of the most profound aspects of genetics in pain perception is its potential to predispose individuals to chronic pain conditions. Chronic pain often arises from an initial injury or illness, but genetic factors can make some people more likely to develop long-term pain.

For example, individuals with a genetic predisposition to higher sensitivity to pain may experience pain more intensely following an injury, and that discomfort may persist long after the injury heals.

Genetic factors can contribute to the development of conditions like:

- **Fibromyalgia:** A chronic pain disorder characterized by widespread pain and tenderness.
- **Osteoarthritis:** A degenerative joint disease where the body's response to joint damage can be exacerbated by genetic factors.
- **Neuropathic Pain:** Pain caused by nerve damage, which can sometimes have a genetic link, particularly in inherited conditions like diabetic neuropathy.

For these patients, pain doesn't necessarily correlate with the extent of physical damage. Instead, the body's pain processing system is hyperactive due to genetic factors, leading to a persistent pain experience.

Genetics and Pain Treatment Response

Genetics also plays a critical role in how well we respond to pain treatments. For example, some people metabolize pain medications faster than others, meaning they may need higher doses to achieve the same effect. On the other hand, some genetic profiles may make individuals more sensitive to certain drugs, making them more prone to side effects or addiction.

The growing field of pharmacogenetics is studying these genetic variations to help tailor pain treatments to individuals. By identifying genetic factors that affect drug metabolism or pain sensitivity, doctors can prescribe more personalized treatment plans, minimizing the trial-and-error approach that many patients experience with pain medications.

Pain and Mental Health: The Genetic Connection

The relationship between genetics, pain, and mental health is also incredibly important. Research has shown that people with certain genetic variations may be more prone to developing anxiety, depression, or other psychological conditions, which can, in turn, heighten their pain perception.

The **COMT gene**, for example, is involved in the breakdown of dopamine, a neurotransmitter linked to mood regulation. Variations in this gene have been associated with a lower threshold for pain, pain as well as a higher risk for anxiety and depression. This makes sense because chronic pain and mental health conditions often coexist, each amplifying the other.

When treating patients with chronic pain, it's crucial to consider both the genetic predispositions for pain and the potential mental health impact. Often, a comprehensive treatment plan that includes both physical and psychological support is necessary.

Genetics and the Future of Pain Management

As our understanding of genetics and pain perception advances, we're moving toward a future where pain management can be more precisely tailored to the individual. With advancements in genetic testing, we may soon be able to predict who is at higher risk for developing chronic pain and customize treatments to prevent or manage it effectively.

For patients, this means the possibility of more targeted, effective treatments with fewer side effects. For doctors, it means being able to create a more personalized pain management plan based on a patient's genetic makeup rather than relying on generalized treatments.

Conclusion

While genetics undoubtedly plays a significant role in how we experience pain, it is important to remember that it is multifaceted Your lifestyle, environment, and even mindset influence your pain, not just your genes. Understanding the role of genetics can help us better approach pain by offering more personalized treatment plans and empowering both doctors and patients to manage it more effectively.

1.5 Societal Stigma Surrounding Chronic Pain

Even those who suffer from chronic pain often misunderstand it. Society's perception of pain is largely shaped by immediate, visible injuries or conditions, such as a broken bone or a burn. We can easily recognize these tangible, physical signs of suffering. But chronic pain is different. It is invisible, persistent, and often difficult to explain. Because of this, it frequently faces societal stigma—misconceptions, judgment, and a lack of empathy that can deeply affect those who live with it every day.

The Invisible Nature of Chronic Pain

One of the most significant challenges faced by individuals with chronic pain is the fact that their suffering isn't visible. When someone walks into a room with a cast or uses a wheelchair, people immediately understand that they are in pain or dealing with an injury. However, someone with chronic pain may look perfectly healthy on the outside, even though they are struggling with severe discomfort.

This invisibility leads to skepticismskepticalness.If they can't see the pain, others may think the person is exaggerating or melodramatic. Unfortunately, this skepticism often leads to the dismissal of the pain as "all in the mind" or as a sign of weakness.

Misunderstanding Pain's Complcxity

Chronic pain is not merely about the physical sensation of discomfort. It involves complex interactions between the nervous system, brain, and psychological state. Yet, society tends to oversimplify the experience of pain, often reducing it to just a physical issue. This misunderstanding fuels the stigma, as people struggle to grasp the deeper, multifaceted nature of pain that extends beyond what they can see.

For many, the assumption is that pain will simply go away with time, or that it's something one can "just get over." The concept of chronic pain, especially when it persists for months or years, is difficult for many to grasp. This lack of understanding leads to feelings of isolation and frustration among those who live with chronic pain every day.

The "Drug Seeker" Stereotype

Another aspect of societal stigma revolves around the treatment of pain, particularly the use of prescription medications. In the past, the opioid crisis has created an unfortunate connection between chronic pain management and drug misuse. As a result, many people with legitimate pain find themselves facing a "drug seeker" stereotype.

People who are prescribed painkillers are sometimes suspected of trying to get high or using them recreationally. This can lead to a lack of proper pain management, as doctors may hesitate to prescribe what they know their patients need, need for fear of being associated with misuse.

This stereotype not only damages trust between patients and healthcare providers but also exacerbates the feelings of alienation that those with chronic pain already experience. For patients, it means enduring their pain in silence, often without the relief they need to function normally in their daily lives.

Social Media and Chronic Pain

In today's age of social media, the pressure to present a perfect life can worsen the stigma surrounding chronic pain. People are constantly posting about their achievements, travels, and milestones, while those with chronic pain often struggle just to get out of bed or go to work. The constant stream of "healthy" and "perfect" images can make those with chronic pain feel even more isolated, as if they're failing to meet societal expectations of well-being.

Moreover, dismissive comments often greet those who share their experiences with chronic pain on platforms like Instagram or Twitter. Phrases like "just get over it" or "everyone gets aches and pains" trivialize the very real and debilitating impact chronic pain can have on a person's life. The lack of empathy and understanding on these platforms further deepens the societal stigma.

Mental Health and Chronic Pain

The stigma associated with mental health often exacerbates the stigma surrounding chronic pain. Many individuals with chronic pain also suffer from depression, anxiety, or other psychological issues. This intersection of physical and mental health issues can create an overwhelming sense of shame and guilt.

People with chronic pain may feel that their emotional struggles are perceived as a weakness or as "not real" because others believe pain should be entirely physical. This lack of understanding can lead to patients suffering in silence, afraid to seek help for both their pain and their mental health.

Breaking the Stigma: A Call for Empathy and Education

The societal stigma surrounding chronic pain is not just a burden on those who suffer from it—it also perpetuates the cycle of misunderstanding and inadequate treatment. The first step in breaking this stigma is through education.

By educating the public about the complexity of chronic pain, we can foster a more compassionate and empathetic society. Chronic pain is not a weakness; it is a medical condition that requires understanding, support, and effective management.

Healthcare professionals also have a crucial role to play in breaking the stigma. By listening to patients without judgment and treating them with respect and diligence, doctors can help create a safe space for patients to talk openly about their pain without fear of being dismissed.

Conclusion

Societal stigma surrounding chronic pain adds an invisible layer of difficulty for those already facing immense physical and emotional challenges. By recognizing the complexity of pain and offering empathy, we can help reduce the isolation and frustration that many with chronic pain endure. Change the narrative, transcend stereotypes, and establish a society that acknowledges, comprehends, and treats pain with the dignity it merits.

Chapter - 2

Exploring The Spectrum Of Pain

2.1 Pain Across Cultures: Global Perspectives

Cultures significantly vary in their understanding, expression, and treatment of pain, despite it being a universal experience. While pain is inherently subjective and shaped by an individual's physical state, emotional response, and personal history, the way society interprets and responds to it is influenced by cultural norms, values, and traditions.In this chapter, we will explore how different cultures perceive pain, how this shapes their treatment approaches, and the societal expectations that govern pain expression.

Cultural Views on Pain: An Overview

Cultural beliefs and societal expectations deeply influence how people experience and interpret pain Many Western societies, especially those that prioritize individualism, often view pain as a personal experience that requires repair or elimination. Medical professionals are often seen as the primary solution providers, with an emphasis on using technology, medication, or surgery to address the source of the pain A biomedical model, which focuses on diagnosing and treating the physical cause of pain, forms the foundation of this mindset.

However, many non-Western cultures view pain from a more holistic perspective. Here, the connection between the mind, body, and spirit is emphasized, and pain is often considered a signal of imbalance, not just a symptom to be removed. Healing may involve physical treatments, but it can also include spiritual, emotional, and communal elements. In these cultures, pain is sometimes viewed as a natural part of life—something to endure and transcend rather than eliminate entirely.

Eastern Traditions: Pain as a Path to Healing

Eastern cultures, especially in countries like China and India, often perceive pain as a manifestation of a deeper imbalance within the body. Traditional healing systems like Traditional Chinese Medicine (TCM) and Ayurveda emphasize the interconnectedness of the body and mind. These systems propose that pain arises when the body's energy—known as "Qi" in Chinese medicine or "Prana" in Ayurveda—is blocked or disrupted.

For example, in TCM, the treatment of pain involves not just addressing the physical symptoms but also restoring the flow of Qi through acupuncture, herbal remedies, and lifestyle adjustments. Pain is not simply a thing to be "fixed" but a signal that something deeper needs attention—whether it's a blockage of energy, an emotional imbalance, or an issue with the body's internal organs.

Similarly, Ayurveda views pain as a symptom of disharmony within the body's three doshas—Vata, Pitta, and Kapha. For the body to function optimally, it is necessary to balance these energies. Pain, from this perspective, serves as an indicator that one or more of the doshas is out of balance, and healing involves addressing the root cause through diet, herbal treatments, yoga, and meditation.

Indigenous Approaches: Pain and Community

Indigenous cultures around the world often have a communal approach to pain, viewing it not just as an individual experience but as something that affects the entire group. Many Indigenous communities understand pain in the context of their spiritual beliefs and communal practices. For instance, certain Native American tribes often view physical pain as a challenge or a milestone, emphasizing the importance of enduring suffering to acquire wisdom and spiritual strength.

In these cultures, healing is often a collective process. Traditional healers, shamans, or spiritual leaders play a crucial role in not only addressing the physical pain but also providing spiritual guidanceThe concept posits a profound connection between emotional and spiritual health and physical well-being Individuals often use rituals, ceremonies, and group support to cope with pain, highlighting the crucial role of the community in the healing process.

Western Approaches: The Biomedical Model of Pain

In contrast, Western medicine often adopts a more individualized, biomedical approach to pain. In this context, physicians often view pain as a symptom of a physiological issue necessitating medical intervention. The focus is on diagnosing the specific cause of the pain, whether it's an injury, illness, or disease, and then treating it with medication, surgery, or other medical procedures.

This model has its advantages, especially when dealing with acute pain resulting from trauma or injury. However, it has limitations when it comes to chronic pain, which often doesn't have a clear, identifiable cause and may persist long after physical healing has occurred. In these cases, pain may be treated with painkillers, nerve blockers, or surgical procedures, but the focus is usually on alleviating symptoms rather than addressing the broader, holistic factors that contribute to the pain experience.

Moreover, the biomedical model often emphasizes a "quick fix" mentality, which can lead to frustration and a sense of helplessness for those dealing with chronic pain. The focus on symptom relief can sometimes overshadow the emotional, psychological, and social components of pain, which can leave patients feeling isolated and misunderstood.

Cultural Attitudes Towards Pain Management

Attitudes toward medical intervention also shape how cultures approach pain management.In many Western societies, there is a greater reliance on pharmaceutical treatments and advanced medical technologies, such as surgery, to address pain. In contrast, other cultures place more value on natural remedies, spiritual healing, and alternative therapies.

In countries like Japan, for example, there is a significant focus on self-care and preventive measures. Pain management often incorporates practices such as Shiatsu massage, herbal medicine, and mindful meditation.In the Mediterranean region, the use of olive oil, herbal infusions, and warm baths is common, reflecting a long-standing cultural connection between health and nature.

Moreover, some cultures may view pain as something that one should quietly endure, even in the face of significant suffering. Cultural concepts of stoicism, self-reliance, and the belief that enduring pain is a sign of strength or moral character often link to this.In contrast, other cultures may encourage more open expression of pain and a willingness to seek help from family, community, or medical professionals.

Globalization and the Sharing of Pain Management Practices

With globalization, there has been a growing exchange of medical knowledge and practices across cultures. Western medicine has incorporated some elements of Eastern and Indigenous practices, such as acupuncture, mindfulness, and herbal remedies, into mainstream pain management. This blending of practices has led to a more integrated approach to pain management, combining the strengths of both traditional and modern treatments.

For example, acupuncture, once seen as a niche treatment, is now widely recognized as an effective therapy for certain types of pain, including back pain and osteoarthritis. Similarly, mindfulness-based stress reduction (MBSR), which originated in Eastern traditions, has gained popularity in the West as an effective tool for managing chronic pain, particularly by helping patients cope with the psychological aspects of their suffering.

Conclusion

Understanding, expressing, and treating pain varies widely across cultures, despite it being a deeply personal and universal experience. Each cultural perspective offers valuable insights into how pain can be managed and alleviated, whether through medical interventions, spiritual practices, or community support. As healthcare professionals, it's essential to recognize and respect the cultural differences in how pain is perceived and treated, as this can greatly influence the effectiveness of treatment. By embracing a more global perspective on pain, we can develop a more holistic and compassionate approach to pain management that addresses both the physical and emotional needs of patients worldwide.

2.2 Pain in the Workplace: An Underestimated Epidemic

Pain in the workplace is a widespread issue, often overlooked, yet it significantly impacts both employees and employers alike. The physical and emotional toll of chronic pain, combined with the pressures of work-related stress, creates a silent epidemic that affects millions worldwide. From office workers to manual laborers, pain is not only a personal health challenge but also a productivity and economic issue that extends far beyond individual suffering.

The Scope of the Problem

Workplace-related pain is not just limited to injuries sustained on the job but also includes musculoskeletal disorders, stress-induced pain, and chronic conditions exacerbated by job demands. Studies have shown that more than 50% of the global workforce experiences some form of work-related pain, with musculoskeletal disorders (MSDs) being the most prevalent. These conditions, including back pain, neck pain, repetitive strain injuries (RSIs), and carpal tunnel syndrome, are responsible for millions of lost workdays each year.

Additionally, pain stemming from emotional and psychological stress—often linked to long hours, heavy workloads, and poor work-life balance—has also become a significant concern. This type of pain, while not always visible, can be just as debilitating as physical pain, leading to mental exhaustion, burnout, and reduced overall well-being.

The Cost of Pain in the Workplace

The cost of pain in the workplace is staggering. According to the World Health Organization (WHO), musculoskeletal disorders alone account for billions of dollars in lost productivity annually. Employees who experience chronic pain are more likely to take sick leave, work fewer hours, or exhibit reduced performance on the job. Pain can also lead to higher rates of absenteeism, presenteeism (when employees are present but working at a reduced capacity), and turnover, all of which come at a substantial cost to businesses.

For employers, the financial burden of workplace pain extends beyond direct medical costs to include lost productivity, workplace accommodations, and the recruitment and training of replacement workers. The economic impact is particularly significant in industries that rely on manual labor, healthcare, or office-based work, where repetitive tasks or poor ergonomics can lead to chronic conditions.

The Physical Toll: Musculoskeletal Disorders (MSDs)

Musculoskeletal disorders (MSDs), which affect the muscles, joints, tendons, ligaments, and nerves, are one of the most common forms of workplace pain. The modern workplace, particularly in office settings, often requires employees to spend long hours sitting at desks, using computers, and performing repetitive motions. Over time, this can lead to discomfort, strain, and permanent damage if not addressed.

For example, prolonged sitting can contribute to lower back pain, while typing for extended periods can cause neck and wrist pain. Poor posture, improper workstation setup, and insufficient breaks can all contribute to MSDs. Even small adjustments, such as using ergonomic furniture or taking regular breaks, can make a significant difference in reducing pain and preventing injury.

In manual labor industries, workers are often at risk of developing pain from physically demanding tasks. Heavy lifting, repetitive movements, and awkward postures can lead to back, shoulder, and joint pain. In these environments, the risk is often higher due to a lack of proper training, inadequate safety measures, or insufficient protective equipment.

The Emotional and Psychological Toll: Stress and Burnout

While physical pain in the workplace is a major concern, emotional and psychological pain is equally, if not more, pervasive. Chronic stress, anxiety, and depression are common among employees in high-pressure work environments. Long hours, demanding deadlines, lack of job security, and workplace conflicts contribute to mental exhaustion, which can manifest as physical pain in the form of headaches, muscle tension, and fatigue.

Stress-induced pain is often referred to as "psychosomatic pain," where the mind and body are interconnected in the experience of discomfort. Emotional pain, such as the stress of managing a heavy workload or feeling unsupported in the workplace, can lead to physical symptoms like muscle aches, digestive issues, and headaches. Over time, this can create a cycle of stress and pain that is difficult to break without intervention.

Today's fast-paced work culture is increasingly concerned about burnout, a state of emotional, physical, and mental exhaustion resulting from excessive and prolonged stress. Employees suffering from burnout are more likely to experience chronic pain, reduced job satisfaction, and diminished quality of life.

The Hidden Impact of Pain on Performance

Pain in the workplace is not always visible, and often, employees will push through the discomfort without seeking help. This "hidden" pain can be incredibly detrimental to both the employee and the company. Many workers endure their pain in silence, refraining from discussing it for fear of appearing weak or unproductive. As a result, they may continue to work despite their discomfort, often leading to worse outcomes in terms of both their health and their job performance.

Presenteeism is a term used to describe employees who are physically present at work but unable to perform at their usual level due to pain, fatigue, or emotional distress. Research has shown that presenteeism can be more costly to businesses than absenteeism, as employees who are working at less than full capacity still incur costs without contributing fully to the organization's productivity.

Additionally, pain often impacts cognitive functions, such as concentration, memory, and decision-making. Employees who are dealing with chronic pain may struggle to focus on tasks, make mistakes, or find it difficult to stay engaged with their work. This leads to lower overall performance, which can have a ripple effect on the company's productivity and success.

Addressing Pain in the Workplace: Solutions and Strategies

To address the growing issue of workplace pain, both employers and employees must take proactive steps. For employers, this involves creating a supportive environment that acknowledges the impact of pain and offers resources for relief. This could include implementing ergonomic workstations, encouraging regular breaks, and providing access to health and wellness programs.

Offering mental health support, such as counseling services, stress management workshops, and fostering a culture that prioritizes mental health, can also benefit workplaces. Employee wellness programs that promote physical activity, relaxation techniques, and mindfulness can help prevent and alleviate stress-related pain.

For employees, it's important to advocate for one's own health and seek help when needed. This means not only addressing physical discomfort but also taking steps to manage stress and emotional pain. Open communication with managers and coworkers about the challenges of dealing with pain can lead to better support and accommodations.

Conclusion

Often underestimated, pain in the workplace has a profound impact on both employees and employers. Chronic pain, whether physical or emotional, can affect productivity, job satisfaction, and overall well-being. By acknowledging the prevalence of workplace pain and creating supportive environments, both organizations and employees can work together to mitigate its effects. A holistic approach to pain management—addressing both the physical and emotional aspects of pain—can lead to healthier, more productive work environments, benefiting everyone involved.

2.3 The Role of Chronic Inflammation

Chronic inflammation is an underlying factor in many painful conditions, yet it is often an invisible and misunderstood process. Unlike acute inflammation, which is the body's natural response to injury or infection and typically resolves once the threat is eliminated, chronic inflammation persists over time. It can silently cause havoc within the body, contributing to a variety of conditions such as joint pain, autoimmune diseases, cardiovascular disease, and even cancer. Understanding chronic inflammation is crucial in managing pain, especially for those suffering from conditions like osteoarthritis, fibromyalgia, or chronic back pain. Inflammation plays a significant role in both the development and progression of the disease.In fact, chronic inflammation is one of the most common and powerful contributors to long-term pain, affecting individuals in ways that are often difficult to recognize or diagnose.

The Mechanisms of Chronic Inflammation

Inflammation is a natural response of the immune system to harmful stimuli such as pathogens, injury, or toxins. When the body encounters these threats, it releases various chemicals, including cytokines and prostaglandins, to protect tissues and fight infection.

However, when the immune system is overstimulated or becomes dysregulated, inflammation can persist, turning into a chronic state.

In chronic inflammation, the body's immune cells continue to produce inflammatory molecules even in the absence of an acute injury or infection. This prolonged inflammation leads to the breakdown of tissues, cartilage, and bones, especially in areas like the joints, which can cause chronic pain and irreversible damage. The body's own cells, in an attempt to repair the damage, can inadvertently cause further harm, perpetuating a vicious cycle of inflammation and pain.

One of the key factors that sustain chronic inflammation is the activation of a group of immune system cells called macrophages. These cells not only protect the body from pathogens but also trigger the release of other inflammatory molecules that can damage surrounding tissue. Over time, the continual activation of these immune cells results in sustained inflammation and ongoing pain.

Inflammation and Pain: The Interconnectedness

There is a close relationship between pain and inflammation. Inflammatory molecules, such as prostaglandins, sensitize the nerves around an inflamed area, amplifying the sensation of pain. This is particularly evident in joint-related pain conditions like rheumatoid arthritis and osteoarthritis, where the inflammation in the joints can lead to increased sensitivity in the surrounding nerves, making even minor movements feel painful.

What makes chronic inflammation particularly problematic is its ability to "reset" the pain response. In an acute injury, pain is a helpful signal that prompts us to protect the affected area and seek treatment. However, in the case of chronic inflammation, pain becomes a constant presence that no longer serves a protective purpose. Instead, it can become a condition in and of itself, making the body more sensitive to pain stimuli even in the absence of a new injury.

Chronic Inflammation in common pain conditions

Chronic inflammation directly links to many common pain conditions or example, in **osteoarthritis**, the wear and tear of cartilage in the joints is often accompanied by low-level inflammation, which exacerbates pain and stiffness. Similarly, **rheumatoid arthritis**, an autoimmune disease, causes the body's immune system to attack its own tissues, leading to inflammation in the joints, which results in debilitating pain and swelling.

Researchers have discovered that low-grade inflammation in the central nervous system may contribute to the heightened pain sensitivity experienced by patients. Despite the ongoing study of the exact mechanisms, it is evident that inflammation significantly influences the perception of pain in these conditions. **Chronic back pain** can also be a result of inflammation. Degenerative disc disease, herniated discs, or spinal stenosis often trigger an inflammatory response in the tissues surrounding the spine, leading to persistent pain. These conditions often elevate inflammatory cytokines, which can intensify the pain, disrupt the healing process, and contribute to long-term discomfort.

Lifestyle Factors That Worsen Chronic Inflammation

Several lifestyle factors can contribute to or exacerbate chronic inflammation, making it important to recognize their role in the pain experience. **Diet** is one of the most significant factors in managing inflammation. Diets high in processed foods, sugars, trans fats, and refined carbohydrates can promote the release of pro-inflammatory molecules in the body. On the other hand, anti-inflammatory foods such as omega-3 fatty acids, antioxidants, and fiber-rich fruits and vegetables have been shown to reduce inflammation and alleviate pain.

Stress also plays a critical role in chronic inflammation. When the body is stressed, it releases stress hormones like cortisol, which, over time, can become less effective in managing inflammation. Chronic stress activates the immune system and triggers the release of inflammatory cytokines, leading to an ongoing cycle of inflammation and pain.

Lack of **exercise** or physical inactivity can further aggravate inflammation. Regular, moderate physical activity has shown to reduce systemic inflammation and decrease pain, while intense or unbalanced exercise can cause temporary inflammation. Conversely, inactivity can lead to an increase in the body's inflammatory markers, especially in those with musculoskeletal pain conditions.

Managing Chronic Inflammation and Pain

To manage chronic inflammation effectively, it's essential to take a holistic approach that combines medical interventions with lifestyle adjustments. Anti-inflammatory medications, such as nonsteroidal anti-inflammatory drugs (NSAIDs), can provide short-term relief from inflammation-related pain. However, due to potential side effects, one should not rely on these for long-term management.

For a more sustainable approach, individuals should consider **dietary changes**, incorporating anti-inflammatory foods, such as fatty fish, nuts, seeds, and leafy greens, into their meals. Supplements, like turmeric or omega-3 fatty acids, may also help reduce inflammation and alleviate pain.

Exercise is another powerful tool in managing chronic inflammation. Low-impact exercises such as swimming, walking, or yoga can improve flexibility, strengthen muscles, and reduce inflammation. These activities also stimulate the production of natural anti-inflammatory substances in the body, which can help mitigate pain.

For those experiencing chronic pain due to inflammation, **stress management techniques** like mindfulness, meditation, and deep breathing exercises can help reduce the release of pro-inflammatory hormones and provide relief from pain. Studies have demonstrated the effectiveness of cognitive-behavioral therapy (CBT) in teaching individuals coping strategies to manage pain, reduce stress, and enhance emotional well-being.

Conclusion

Chronic inflammation is a major driver of persistent pain and is often at the heart of many chronic conditions. Its ability to fuel both physical and emotional suffering makes it a significant obstacle to pain relief and recovery. However, by understanding the role of inflammation in the body, making lifestyle changes, and pursuing appropriate treatments, individuals can better manage the pain it causes.

Taking a proactive approach to managing inflammation is crucial in improving quality of life and regaining control over one's health.

2.4 Pediatric Pain: An Overlooked Challenge

People often underestimate, misunderstand, or dismiss pain in children. Unlike adults, who can articulate their pain and describe its intensity and location, children have limited ability to express what they are feeling. This gap in communication, combined with a lack of awareness about pediatric pain, can lead to delayed diagnoses, inadequate treatment, and a lack of proper pain management. Unfortunately, pediatric pain remains one of the most overlooked and under addressed challenges in medicine, and it is critical that we change this perception.

Pain in children can arise from a variety of causes, including injuries, chronic conditions, infections, surgeries, or even psychological stress. Whether it's a simple headache, growing pains, or the acute pain from a broken bone, the experience of pain in a child can have profound effects on their physical and emotional well-being. In many cases, pain can interfere with their ability to engage in normal daily activities, such as playing, going to school, or even sleeping. Moreover, unresolved pain can lead to longer-term consequences, including the development of chronic pain conditions that persist into adulthood.

The Complexity of Pediatric Pain

One of the greatest challenges in managing pediatric pain is the subjective nature of pain itself. Children, especially those who are very young or have limited verbal skills, often struggle to communicate how much pain they are in or where they feel it. This makes it difficult for healthcare providers to assess the severity of the pain and, more importantly, to determine the appropriate treatment plan.

Additionally, children may express their pain through behavior, such as crying, irritability, or changes in appetite or sleep patterns. In some cases, they may withdraw from social activities or exhibit signs of anxiety or depression. People often overlook or misinterpret these non-verbal cues, which can result in treatment delays or incorrect diagnoses. Even when children can communicate their pain, the language they use may be vague or inconsistent, further complicating the situation.

There is also the issue of **developmental differences** in how children experience and respond to pain. Younger children may not have developed the cognitive or emotional coping mechanisms to handle pain as well as older children or adults. As a result, they may experience heightened distress or fear, which can amplify their pain perception. Moreover, children's brains are still developing, and repeated exposure to pain during this critical time can alter the way their nervous systems process and respond to pain in the future.

The Impact of Chronic Pain in Children

Chronic pain is particularly concerning when it affects children, as it can severely disrupt their physical, emotional, and social development. Conditions such as **juvenile arthritis**, **migraine headaches**, **sickle cell disease**, and **fibromyalgia** can cause persistent, recurring pain that can last for months or even years. These conditions not only affect the child's quality of life but can also interfere with their academic performance, friendships, and family life.

Children living with chronic pain often experience a cascade of negative outcomes. Pain can lead to **sleep disturbances**, which in turn affect mood, concentration, and cognitive function. It can cause children to become more sedentary, as physical activity may worsen their pain, leading to a decline in overall health. In the long run, chronic pain can contribute to **emotional distress**, including anxiety, depression, and feelings of isolation. Furthermore, the longer a child experiences untreated pain, the more likely they are to develop **a pain-related disability** that persists into adulthood.

The Importance of Early Intervention

Early recognition and treatment of pain in children are critical to preventing long-term consequences. Taking pediatric pain seriously is the first step in addressing it.

Healthcare providers must learn to recognize the signs of pain, even when they are not directly expressed, and should always consider pain as a potential cause when a child presents with behavioral or physical symptoms.

In the case of **acute pain**, such as pain from an injury or surgery, the goal is to manage the pain promptly and effectively, preventing it from transitioning into chronic pain. This may involve the use of **analgesics** (pain relievers), **anti-inflammatory medications**, and **topical treatments**, along with psychological techniques like **relaxation exercises** and **distraction methods** to help children cope with pain.

When dealing with **chronic pain**, the approach becomes more complex, as the pain may have both physical and psychological components. Treating chronic pediatric pain requires a multidisciplinary approach, including medical management, physical therapy, psychological support, and education for both the child and their family. Research has demonstrated the effectiveness of cognitive-behavioral therapy (CBT) in assisting children in managing the emotional distress associated with chronic pain. This form of therapy helps children develop positive coping mechanisms and understand the connection between their thoughts, emotions, and pain.

The Role of Parents and Caregivers

Parents and caregivers play a crucial role in managing pediatric pain. Their ability to recognize pain, provide emotional support, and ensure that the child adheres to treatment plans is essential. Often, parents are the ones who observe changes in their child's behavior and seek medical attention. Therefore, it's crucial to educate parents about pain management strategies and empower them to advocate for their child's needs.

Parents should be encouraged to help their child develop **self-care skills**, such as relaxation techniques, proper posture, and understanding their pain triggers. Additionally, it's important for parents to provide emotional reassurance and ensure that their child feels supported throughout their pain management journey. Encouraging a child to remain active, despite their pain, can also help prevent the physical deconditioning that often accompanies chronic pain.

The Psychological Aspect of Pediatric Pain

Emotional and psychological factors deeply entwine with pain, making it more than just a physical sensation. Children experiencing pain may also experience fear, anxiety, frustration, and sadness, which can amplify their experience. For example, children with chronic pain may become anxious about engaging in normal activities or worry about future pain episodes. This emotional distress can create a feedback loop, where anxiety increases the perception of pain, and pain increases anxiety.

Incorporating psychological support into pain management is essential for children suffering from persistent or chronic pain. Techniques such as **mindfulness**, **relaxation training**, and **guided imagery** can help children break the cycle of pain and anxiety. Family therapy may also be beneficial, especially in cases where the pain has significantly impacted family dynamics.

A Multidisciplinary Approach to Pediatric Pain

The most effective treatment for pediatric pain is a **multidisciplinary approach** that incorporates medical, psychological, and educational interventions. Pediatric pain specialists, physical therapists, psychologists, and primary care doctors must work together to create a comprehensive treatment plan tailored to the child's individual needs.

This approach should also include education for the child and their family, as understanding the nature of the pain and the treatment options can empower both the child and the caregivers.It is important to approach pediatric pain from a holistic perspective, recognizing that it affects not only the body but also the mind and the child's overall development.

Conclusion

Pediatric pain is a serious and often overlooked issue that deserves more attention and research. Pain in children, whether acute or chronic, can significantly affect their development, emotional well-being, and quality of life. By recognizing the signs of pain early, providing comprehensive treatment, and involving both medical professionals and caregivers in the process, we can help ensure that children experience the best possible outcomes. Pain management necessitates a personalized approach that takes into account the unique needs of each child.

Chapter - 3

Advances In Understanding Pain

3.1 Precision Medicine: Customizing Pain Relief

The concept of precision medicine has revolutionized many aspects of healthcare, and its application in pain management holds enormous promise. Unlike the traditional "one-size-fits-all" approach, precision medicine focuses on tailoring treatment to the individual characteristics of each patient, including their genetic makeup, environment, lifestyle, and the specific nature of their pain. This approach allows for a more targeted and effective pain management strategy, leading to improved outcomes and fewer side effects.

Pain is a complex, multifaceted phenomenon that varies greatly from person to person. While two individuals might experience the same condition—say, osteoarthritis—they may perceive and respond to pain in completely different ways. One might suffer from intense, constant pain, while the other might experience intermittent discomfort. This variability is due to a combination of biological, psychological, and social factors, which is why a personalized approach to pain relief is so essential.

Precision medicine integrates a range of advanced techniques and technologies to better understand these individual differences and customize treatment. By focusing on the underlying causes of pain rather than just treating its symptoms, it offers the potential for more effective and sustainable pain relief.

The Role of Genetics in Precision Pain Management

One of the foundational principles of precision medicine is understanding the role of **genetics** in pain perception. Each person's genetic makeup influences how they experience and process pain. Certain genes can make some individuals more susceptible to chronic pain, while others might have a higher pain threshold. For example, variations in genes that affect the **opioid receptors** in the brain can influence how an individual responds to painkillers like morphine. Similarly, mutations in **inflammatory pathways** can determine how the body reacts to conditions like rheumatoid arthritis or back pain.

Advances in **genomic sequencing** now allow doctors to assess a patient's genetic profile and identify specific pain-related gene variations. This information can help predict how a person will respond to different treatments, including medications and therapies. For instance, if a person has a genetic predisposition to metabolize certain pain medications more slowly, a doctor can adjust the dosage to avoid side effects or ineffectiveness. Similarly, by understanding genetic variations in pain sensitivity, doctors can identify the most appropriate pain management strategy, minimizing the trial-and-error process that often comes with traditional treatment approaches.

Personalized Treatment Plans

Another key component of precision medicine in pain management is the development of **personalized treatment plans** that take into account not just genetics but also the patient's lifestyle, environment, and psychological state. Factors such as stress, poor sleep, sedentary behavior, and mental health conditions like anxiety and depression often exacerbate chronic pain. Understanding these variables allows doctors to create comprehensive treatment plans that address all aspects of a patient's health.

For example, a personalized plan for someone suffering from chronic lower back pain might include a combination of physical therapy, medications, stress-reducing techniques such as **mindfulness**, and perhaps even dietary changes that reduce inflammation. Precision medicine enables healthcare providers to combine these elements in ways that are specifically tailored to the individual patient's unique needs.

Another aspect of this approach involves using **biomarkers**—biological indicators that can provide information about the underlying causes of pain. By analyzing blood tests, imaging results, and even the body's response to certain medications, doctors can pinpoint which treatments are most likely to provide relief. This helps avoid the trial-and-error process that is often frustrating for patients and can lead to prolonged suffering.

Technological Advancements in Precision Pain Management

In recent years, technology has played a major role in advancing precision medicine for pain relief. Innovations in **neuroimaging** and **electrodiagnostic testing** have made it easier to identify the exact source of pain and monitor how it responds to different treatments. Doctors can observe brain activity in real-time using techniques like functional MRI (fMRI), which aids in their understanding of how the brain processes pain signals. This information can be used to adjust treatment strategies in a way that is more precisely aligned with the patient's individual pain pathways.

Similarly, **genetic testing** and **pharmacogenomics**—the study of how genes affect a person's response to drugs—are enabling healthcare providers to prescribe medications that are more effective and less likely to cause adverse reactions. For example, certain medications may not work for individuals with specific gene mutations, and understanding this can help doctors avoid ineffective treatments. As our knowledge of pharmacogenomics expands, doctors will be able to offer even more targeted drug regimens that provide better pain relief with fewer side effects.

In addition, **wearable devices** are emerging as tools for managing and personalizing pain relief. These devices can continuously monitor vital signs like heart rate, blood pressure, and muscle tension, providing real-time data to both patients and healthcare providers. This data allows for more dynamic and adaptive pain management, where adjustments can be made on the fly to optimize relief.

Integrating Psychosocial Factors into Precision Pain Medicine

While genetics and technology are crucial in the precision pain management model, we must also acknowledge the **psychosocial** factors that significantly impact a patient's pain experience. Mental health conditions like **depression**, **anxiety**, and **chronic stress** are frequently intertwined with chronic pain, making it more difficult to achieve long-term relief. Precision medicine embraces this aspect by incorporating **psychological assessments** and **therapy** into the treatment plan.

For example, cognitive-behavioral therapy (CBT), mindfulness techniques, and **biofeedback** are often integrated into personalized pain management plans to help patients reframe their perception of pain, manage stress, and build resilience. By considering the patient's emotional state, cognitive patterns, and personal history, healthcare providers can offer more holistic and effective treatment that goes beyond medication alone.

The Future of Precision Pain Management

The future of precision medicine in pain management looks incredibly promising. As technology advances, the ability to track, measure, and analyze pain in realtime will become more sophisticated. Healthcare providers will develop more precise and personalized treatments, resulting in greater efficacy and fewer side effects. The integration of **big data** and **artificial intelligence** into pain management will allow healthcare providers to create highly individualized treatment regimens based on the patient's unique pain profile.

We are also on the cusp of breakthroughs in **regenerative medicine**, where treatments like **stem cell therapy** and **gene editing** could be used to repair or regenerate damaged tissues that cause chronic pain. These advancements may offer permanent solutions for conditions like osteoarthritis, neuropathic pain, and other degenerative diseases.

However, for all its potential, precision medicine must remain accessible and affordable. As we move forward, it will be important to ensure that these advanced treatments are available to patients from all walks of life, not just those who can afford the latest technologies.

Conclusion

Precision medicine is changing the way we understand and treat pain. By focusing on individual differences, incorporating genetic insights, and using advanced technologies, we can customize treatment in a way that was previously unimaginable. This approach promises to offer more effective, sustainable pain relief, reducing the trial-and-error process and improving the quality of life for countless individuals suffering from chronic pain. As we continue to explore this new frontier, the future of pain management appears more promising than ever before.

3.2 Biomarkers for Pain Diagnosis

Pain has long been recognized as a subjective experience—one that varies from person to person, shaped by individual factors such as genetics, environment, and psychological state. Despite this variability, pain has traditionally been assessed based on patients' descriptions of their symptoms, often leading to challenges in accurate diagnosis and treatment. However, recent advancements in pain management have introduced **biomarkers** as a groundbreaking tool for diagnosing and understanding pain with greater precision.

Biomarkers are measurable substances or characteristics in the body that indicate the presence or severity of a disease, condition, or physiological state. In the context of pain, biomarkers can provide objective data that reflect the underlying biological processes involved, offering valuable insights into how pain is experienced, perceived, and managed. The ability to measure pain through biomarkers opens up new opportunities for clinicians to diagnose discomfort more accurately and tailor treatments to individual patients, improving outcomes and reducing the reliance on subjective reports.

Types of Biomarkers in Pain Diagnosis

Biomarkers for pain diagnosis can be categorized into several types, depending on the method of measurement and the biological process being examined. Some of the most significant categories include **inflammatory**

biomarkers, **neurotransmitter biomarkers**, and **genetic biomarkers**.

1. Inflammatory Biomarkers

Chronic pain is often associated with **inflammation**, particularly in conditions such as arthritis, fibromyalgia, and neuropathy. Inflammation can cause or exacerbate pain by sensitizing nerve endings and promoting the release of chemical substances that heighten the pain response. Measuring **inflammatory biomarkers** can provide clinicians with valuable data about the level of inflammation in the body, which directly correlates with pain severity.

C-reactive protein (CRP), a substance the liver produces in response to inflammation, is one of the most commonly studied inflammatory biomarkers. Elevated levels of CRP are often seen in individuals with chronic pain conditions, making it a potential marker for identifying and monitoring pain related to inflammation. Other substances, such as interleukins (IL-6) and tumor necrosis factor-alpha (TNF-α), are also important in the inflammatory process and may show how bad the pain is or how fast it is getting worse.

For patients with conditions like osteoarthritis or rheumatoid arthritis, measuring these inflammatory biomarkers can help doctors assess how much inflammation is contributing to the pain and whether treatments aimed at reducing it, such as non-steroidal anti-inflammatory drugs (NSAIDs) or biologic agents, will be effective.

2. Neurotransmitter Biomarkers

Neurotransmitters are chemicals that transmit signals in the nervous system, playing a critical role in how pain is perceived. The levels of specific neurotransmitters can influence both the intensity and duration of pain. By measuring neurotransmitter biomarkers, doctors can gain insights into the **central nervous system's (CNS)** role in pain processing and identify potential therapeutic targets.

Substance P, a neuropeptide that nerve cells release in response to injury or inflammation, is an important neurotransmitter involved in pain perception. Substance P, a neuropeptide that nerve cells release in response to injury or inflammation, is an important neurotransmitter involved in pain perception. Glutamate, the primary excitatory neurotransmitter in the brain, plays a crucial role in conditions such as neuropathic pain and migraines.

In addition, **endogenous opioids**, such as **endorphins** and **enkephalins**, are the body's natural pain-relieving substances. A deficiency in these neuropeptides can contribute to chronic pain, and measuring their levels may help clinicians understand the pain mechanisms at play in a particular patient. These biomarkers can also offer insights into why some patients respond well to opioid medications, while others may require alternative treatments.

3. Genetic Biomarkers

Genetic differences can significantly affect how individuals perceive pain and respond to treatments.

Genetic biomarkers offer a personalized approach to pain diagnosis and management by identifying patients who may be at a higher risk for developing chronic pain or who might respond better to certain therapies.

For instance, studies have shown that variations in the OPRM1 gene, which encodes the mu-opioid receptor, influence an individual's sensitivity to opioid medications. Patients with certain variations may experience enhanced pain relief from opioids, while others may have a reduced response In the same way, differences in catechol-O-methyltransferase (COMT), an enzyme that breaks down dopamine, can affect how sensitive you are to pain and your chance of getting fibromyalgia or chronic back pain.

Genetic testing for pain-related biomarkers is still an emerging field, but it holds significant potential for offering more personalized pain management strategies. By understanding a patient's genetic predispositions, doctors can better predict which treatments will be effective and avoid those that might cause unnecessary side effects.

Biomarkers in Clinical Practice

The potential for biomarkers to improve pain diagnosis and management is vast. However, for biomarkers to become a standard tool in clinical practice, they must meet specific criteria. First and foremost, biomarkers must be reliable and valid—meaning they must consistently reflect the presence and severity of pain across diverse patient populations. They also need to be simple to measure using non-invasive methods, such as blood tests, saliva samples, or skin biopsies, so they can be applied in everyday clinical settings.

While researchers are making strides in identifying and validating biomarkers for pain, there are still challenges to overcome before they can be widely used in practice. For instance, the intricate nature of pain necessitates the use of multiple biomarkers to fully encompass its scope. Additionally, there are ethical considerations surrounding the use of genetic testing, as it raises concerns about privacy, consent, and the potential for discrimination.

Despite these challenges, the integration of biomarkers into pain management has the potential to revolutionize the way we diagnose and treat pain. Biomarkers help doctors better tailor treatments, improve patient outcomes, and cut down on the trial-and-error that usually comes with traditional pain management methods. They do this by giving doctors a more objective and precise picture of how pain works.

The Future of Biomarkers in Pain Diagnosis

As research into biomarkers for pain continues to advance, we can expect to see more **sophisticated tests** and **diagnostic tools** emerge. The use of **big data** and **machine learning** is also opening up exciting possibilities for identifying patterns in biomarker data that may not be apparent through traditional methods. For instance, combining genetic, inflammatory, and neurotransmitter biomarkers into a complete diagnostic tool could lead to very personalized pain management plans that make treatment work best for each patient.

The future of pain management lies in the ability to understand pain on a **molecular** level and treat it based on the specific biological processes at play in each individual. With the rise of precision medicine and the growing body of research on pain biomarkers, we are on the verge of a new era in pain relief—one that is more effective, efficient, and personalized than ever before.

3.3 Virtual Reality: A Game-Changer in Pain Therapy

The human experience of pain has always been subjective, personal, and challenging to quantify. Traditional methods of managing pain typically involve medications, physical therapy, or surgical intervention. However, as medical technology advances, new methods of pain relief are being explored, and one of the most exciting developments in recent years has been the use of **Virtualvirtual Realityreality (VR)** in pain management.

Virtual reality, once thought of as a tool solely for gaming and entertainment, is now being recognized as a powerful modality for pain relief, with the potential to alter how we approach pain therapy. By immersing patients in a fully interactive, computer-generated environment, VR has the ability to distract the brain from the sensation of pain, offering an innovative, non-pharmacological alternative to traditional pain relief methods.

How Virtual Reality Works in Pain Therapy

Virtual reality fundamentally modifies the perception of pain by engaging the brainImmersion in a VR environment diverts a patient's attention from their pain through visual, auditory, and even tactile stimuli. This phenomenon is known as **distraction therapy**, and it is based on the concept that pain signals are processed in the brain along with other sensory information.

The brain has limited capacity for processing sensory input at any given time. When a person is fully engaged in an immersive VR experience, the brain focuses on the virtual environment rather than the pain signals being sent from the body. This "distraction" can reduce the perception of pain, as the brain prioritizes the more engaging stimuli of the VR environment over the painful sensations.

Additionally, VR has the potential to directly influence the brain's pain processing mechanisms through a concept known as **neuroplasticity**. By repeatedly exposing patients to immersive, pleasant virtual experiences, VR may help train the brain to reduce its sensitivity to pain over time, potentially leading to long-term pain relief.

Applications of Virtual Reality in Pain Management

Virtual reality has shown tremendous promise in managing a wide range of pain conditions, from acute to chronic pain. Several key applications of VR in pain therapy are beginning to emerge:

1. Acute Pain Relief in Medical Settings

One of the most well-established uses of VR in pain management is in **acute pain relief** for patients undergoing medical procedures, such as wound dressing changes, burn care, or even dental work. In these cases, VR is used to help patients cope with the immediate pain and distress associated with these procedures by providing them with a more enjoyable and engaging experience.

For example, research has shown that burn victims who used VR during painful wound dressing changes reported significantly lower pain levels compared to those who received standard care. VR in these settings can reduce the need for pain medications, particularly opioids, which can carry risks of addiction and side effects.

2. Chronic Pain Management

Chronic pain, which lasts for months or even years, can be incredibly debilitating, with conditions like **fibromyalgia**, **back pain**, and **complex regional pain syndrome (CRPS)** presenting ongoing challenges for both patients and healthcare providers. VR therapy significantly reduces pain intensity, improves mood, and enhances overall quality of life for patients dealing with chronic painVR often serves as a form of mental distraction and relaxation therapy in this context. Patients may be guided through calming virtual environments, such as a serene beach, forest, or garden, which can evoke positive emotions and promote a sense of peace. This relaxation can help counteract the stress and tension that often accompany chronic pain, further reducing pain perception.

3. Neuroplasticity and Pain Rewiring

In addition to its role in distraction, VR has the potential to aid in **neuroplasticity**—the brain's ability to reorganize itself and form new neural connections in response to experience. Certain VR programs have been specifically designed to target the brain's pain processing pathways, providing a form of "therapy" that helps retrain the brain to respond differently to pain.

For example, patients with phantom limb pain—a condition in which amputees experience sensations or pain in a limb that no longer exists—have used VR to "re-map" the brain. Virtual reality (VR) can help with long-term pain management by reducing the frequency and intensity of phantom limb sensations by simulating the movement of the missing limb through virtual feedback.

The Science Behind Virtual Reality's Effectiveness

The effectiveness of VR in pain therapy lies in both **neuroscience** and **psychology**. Neuroscientific studies show that the brain processes pain signals in areas such as the **somatosensory cortex**, which is responsible for processing physical sensations. However, the limbic system and prefrontal cortex process emotional and cognitive aspects of pain, such as fear, anxiety, and frustration.

By immersing patients in a virtual environment, VR stimulates the brain's visual, auditory, and motor pathways, activating different areas of the brain, including those responsible for emotional regulation. This sensory input can help modulate the brain's response to pain by reducing the activation of the pain-related areas and enhancing feelings of control, relaxation, and pleasure.

Moreover, VR can stimulate the release of **endorphins**—the body's natural painkillers—through its effect on the brain's reward system. This neurochemical response further supports VR's potential to reduce pain, offering an additional layer of efficacy.

Limitations and Future Directions Future directions

Virtual reality, despite its promising results, is not a universally applicable solution for pain management. Several factors, including the type of pain, the patient's willingness to engage in VR therapy, and the design of the VR program, influence the effectiveness of the treatment. For some patients, especially those with severe cognitive impairments or extreme pain, VR may not provide significant relief. Furthermore, the cost and accessibility of VR technology can limit its widespread use in certain healthcare settings.

However, the future of VR in pain therapy is promising. More advanced and personalized VR programs, tailored to an individual's unique pain profile, will emerge as technology continues to evolve. New technologies like haptic feedback, which adds tactile sensations to virtual environments, and biofeedback systems that track the patient's body's responses during VR therapy will make the experience even better

In the years to come, VR has the potential to become a cornerstone of pain management, offering a non-invasive, drug-free alternative that can complement traditional therapies and revolutionize the way we treat pain. As we continue to explore its benefits and refine its application, virtual reality has the potential to revolutionize the treatment of both acute and chronic pain.

3.4 Exploring the Gut-Pain Axis

The gut-brain connection has long fascinated scientists, but we only recently began to understand its complexity and importance merging research has revealed an intricate communication network between the **gut** and the **brain** that plays a pivotal role in the sensation and modulation of pain. This interaction, known as the **gut-brain axis**, has profound implications for how we understand and manage chronic pain.

The gut-brain axis is the system of two-way communication between the gastrointestinal (GI) tract and the central nervous system (CNS), which is made up of the brain and spinal cord. This network is not only responsible for regulating digestion but also influences emotional health, immune function, and pain perception. New research shows that this communication pathway may play a part in a number of chronic pain conditions, mainly visceral (pain in the organs), like migraines, irritable bowel syndrome (IBS), and fibromyalgia.

The Science Behind the Gut-Pain Axis

The gut is often referred to as the "second brain" because it contains an extensive network of neurons, known as the **enteric nervous system (ENS)**, which is capable of functioning independently of the central nervous system. But the gut-brain axis is based on the vagus nerve connecting the ENS to the brain. The vagus nerve, one of the largest nerves in the body, acts as a communication highway, transmitting signals in both directions—**from the gut to the brain** and **from the brain to the gut**. Several factors, including gut microbiota (the bacteria and other microorganisms that inhabit our intestines), hormones, immune cells, and neurotransmitters, can influence these signalsAll of these elements contribute to the regulation of pain and discomfort in the body, particularly in the context of chronic pain conditions.

The gut microbiota, microbiota in particular, particular has emerged as a critical player in this complex relationship. The trillions of bacteria in the gut not only aid in digestion but also produce a range of neuroactive substances, including **serotonin**, which is a key regulator of mood and pain perception. Studies have shown that imbalances in the gut microbiota—known as **dysbiosis**—can lead to disruptions in brain function and may exacerbate conditions like chronic pain, anxiety, and depression.

The Role of Gut Health in Chronic Pain Conditions

People increasingly recognize the gut-brain axis as one of the critical contributing factors to chronic pain conditions, which often have a multifactorial origin. The following conditions are particularly influenced by this gut-pain interaction:

1. Irritable Bowel Syndrome (IBS)

IBS is a common gastrointestinal disorder that causes chronic abdominal pain, bloating, and changes in bowel habits. While the precise cause of IBS remains unclear, emerging research suggests that disruptions in the gut-brain axis may be a key factor. Individuals with IBS frequently exhibit increased sensitivity to typical gut sensations, potentially due to alterations in the brain's processing of pain signals. Moreover, patients with IBS frequently report comorbidities such as **anxiety** and **depression**, further suggesting a complex interplay between gut health and emotional wellbeing.

Some researchers believe that **gut dysbiosis**, or an imbalance of gut bacteria, may trigger or exacerbate the symptoms of IBS by affecting the communication between the gut and the brain. Patients may experience pain due to abnormal digestive tract function and brain pain signaling.

2. Fibromyalgia

Fibromyalgia is another chronic pain condition characterized by widespread muscle pain, fatigue, and sleep disturbances. Interestingly, many patients with fibromyalgia also report gastrointestinal issues, including symptoms commonly seen in IBS. Research has shown that individuals with fibromyalgia have altered gut microbiota, which may contribute to both the pain and the GI disturbances experienced by these patients. The pain perception in fibromyalgia may be heightened by abnormal communication between the gut and the brain, resulting in the amplification of pain signals.

3. Migraines

Migraines are intense, recurring headaches often accompanied by symptoms such as nausea and light sensitivity. Emerging research indicates that there may be a connection between gut health and migraine susceptibility. People with migraines are more likely to have GI issues, such as nausea and bloating, and alterations in gut microbiota have been linked to the severity of migraine attacks. The gut-brain axis may play a role in the onset and persistence of migraines, with gut disturbances potentially triggering or amplifying the pain signals that lead to a migraine attack.

The Impact of Gut Dysbiosis on Pain Perception

Dysbiosis refers to an imbalance or disruption in the gut microbiota that can lead to systemic inflammation, immune dysfunction, and altered brain function. This imbalance may be a key factor in the development of chronic pain conditions. In fact, research has shown that certain bacteria in the gut can influence pain processing by altering the levels of pain-related neurotransmitters and immune molecules.

For example, gut-derived short-chain fatty acids (SCFAs), which are produced by gut bacteria's fermentation of fiber, have been shown to have anti-inflammatory effects and may help reduce pain. However, dysbiosis can impair SCFA production, resulting in heightened inflammation and amplified pain signals. In addition, dysbiosis has been linked to **leaky gut syndrome**, where the intestinal lining becomes more permeable, allowing harmful bacteria and toxins to enter the bloodstream. This can trigger systemic inflammation and worsen pain perception.

Managing Pain Through Gut Health

Given the growing understanding of the gut-pain axis, improving gut health may offer a novel strategy for managing chronic pain. Some of the most promising approaches to managing pain through the gut-brain connection include:

1. Probiotics and Prebiotics

Probiotics, which are beneficial bacteria that can be taken as supplements, have shown promise in balancing gut microbiota and improving symptoms of chronic pain, particularly in conditions like IBS. Prebiotics, which are non-digestible fibers that feed healthy gut bacteria, may also help restore balance to the microbiome. Together, probiotics and prebiotics can support a healthier gut environment, potentially reducing inflammation and pain.

2. Diet and Nutrition

A balanced diet rich in **fiber**, **omega-3 fatty acids**, and **anti-inflammatory foods** can promote gut health and support pain management. Avoiding inflammatory foods like processed sugars, refined grains, and trans fats may also help reduce the risk of gut dysbiosis and its associated pain symptoms.

3. Mindfulness and Stress Reduction

Because the gut-brain axis is sensitive to stress, managing emotional and psychological wellbeing is crucial for pain management. Techniques such as **mindfulness meditation**, **yoga**, and **cognitive-behavioral therapy (CBT)** can help reduce stress and inflammation, ultimately improving both gut health and pain perception.

Conclusion: A Holistic Approach to Pain Relief

The gut-pain axis represents a groundbreaking area of research in the field of pain management. By understanding how the gut and brain communicate, we can gain new insights into the causes of chronic pain and develop more effective, holistic treatment approaches. Addressing gut health—through diet, probiotics, stress management, and other interventions—holds promise for improving pain relief and enhancing the overall quality of life for individuals suffering from chronic pain conditions.

As we continue to explore this connection, the future of pain management may increasingly rely on treatments that nurture the delicate balance between the gut and the brain, offering patients more sustainable and comprehensive solutions for managing pain.

3.5 Neuroplasticity and Pain: New Frontiers

The concept of **neuroplasticity**—the brain's ability to reorganize itself by forming new neural connections throughout life—has revolutionized our understanding of the nervous system and its role in chronic pain. We now view what was once believed to be a fixed, unchangeable network as a dynamic, adaptable system.

Neuroplasticity plays a central role in how the brain processes pain, and its implications for pain management are profound. Understanding this concept opens up new frontiers in the way we approach chronic pain treatment, offering hope for those suffering from conditions previously thought to be untreatable.

The Role of Neuroplasticity in Pain

Pain, especially **chronic pain**, is not just a physical sensation; it is a complex neurological experience that involves both **sensory** and **emotional** components. When pain persists beyond the normal healing period, it can undergo a transformation in the brain. Chronic pain can lead to changes in the **central nervous system** (CNS), particularly in areas involved in pain processing, such as the **spinal cord**, **brainstem**, and **cortex**. These changes are a direct result of neuroplasticity, where the brain "learns" to continue perceiving pain even in the absence of an ongoing injury or tissue damage.

How Neuroplasticity Contributes to Chronic Pain

Neuroplasticity presents a complex issue in the realm of pain.

While it can be beneficial for recovery and learning, it can also work against us in the case of chronic pain. Here's how:

1. Central Sensitization

One of the most well-documented phenomena associated with chronic pain is **central sensitization**, where the brain becomes hyper-reactive to pain signals. Normally, the body's pain receptors (nociceptors) send signals to the brain when there is injury or inflammation. However, in cases of chronic pain, these signals can become amplified and misinterpreted, leading to a persistent pain experience. Central sensitization occurs when neural circuits in the CNS become overly responsive due to neuroplastic changes, and the brain starts to "feel" pain even in response to non-painful stimuli.

For example, someone with **fibromyalgia** might experience severe pain from light touch or mild pressure, even though there is no physical cause for such a sensation. People who have chronic pain change the way their brain's neural pathways work, which makes them overly sensitive to pain and disproportionate to the injury.

2. Maladaptive Plasticity

Neuroplasticity can lead to **maladaptive plasticity**, where the brain "learns" to interpret pain signals in ways that are not useful for survival or healing. In chronic pain conditions, the brain's response to pain can become so ingrained that it continues even after the initial cause of pain has resolved. This maladaptive change is not only limited to the sensory components of pain but can also influence the **emotional** and **cognitive** aspects of the pain experience.

For instance, in conditions like **chronic back pain**, the brain may continue to produce pain sensations long after the injury has healed because the neural networks responsible for pain processing have been reinforced and strengthened by repeated pain signals. This continued "learning" of pain makes it more difficult to break the cycle of chronic pain.

3. Pain Memory

The brain can develop a form of "pain memory," where the experience of pain is stored in the neural circuits in a way that becomes deeply entrenched. This memory of pain makes the brain more sensitive to future pain signals and can contribute to the development of **pain catastrophizing**, a psychological response where individuals feel as though their pain will never end or that it is more severe than it truly is. This often leads to increased emotional distress, anxiety, and depression, all of which amplify the pain experience.

Harnessing Neuroplasticity for Pain Relief

While neuroplasticity can contribute to the persistence of chronic pain, it also offers the potential for healing and recovery. By understanding and leveraging the brain's ability to reorganize itself, new therapeutic approaches can be developed that focus on **retraining the brain** and reversing the maladaptive changes that underlie chronic pain.

1. Cognitive Behavioral Therapy (CBT)

One of the most powerful tools in reversing maladaptive neuroplasticity is **cognitive behavioral therapy (CBT)**. CBT focuses on changing the thought patterns and behaviors that contribute to the perception of pain. It can help individuals reframe their understanding of pain, reduce fear and anxiety, and learn how to manage it through coping strategies. Over time, these changes in thinking can lead to physical changes in the brain, helping to reduce the intensity and frequency of pain signals.

By training the brain to respond differently to pain, CBT can help break the cycle of chronic pain, allowing patients to regain control over their lives and reduce reliance on medication.

2. Graded Exposure Therapy

Graded exposure therapy is another form of treatment that utilizes the principles of neuroplasticity. This approach gradually exposes patients to physical activities or movements they have been avoiding due to pain. The goal is to "retrain" the brain to tolerate pain in a controlled and gradual way, essentially rewiring the brain to view these activities as less threatening. As the brain learns that certain movements or actions do not result in pain, the neural pathways associated with pain become weaker, and the pain response diminishes.

This form of therapy is particularly effective for individuals with conditions like **chronic back pain** or **osteoarthritis**, where fear of movement can perpetuate pain.

3. Mindfulness and Meditation

Mindfulness and **meditation** techniques also leverage neuroplasticity by training the brain to focus on the present moment, reduce stress, and develop healthier emotional responses to pain. Regular mindfulness practice can decrease the brain's hyperactivity in areas involved in pain perception and promote a state of relaxation that counteracts pain. Studies have shown that mindfulness can lead to changes in brain structures associated with pain, reducing the brain's sensitivity to pain signals.

By fostering a non-judgmental awareness of pain, mindfulness allows individuals to experience pain without becoming overwhelmed by it, which can lead to significant reductions in the intensity and emotional impact of pain.

4. Physical Therapy and Exercise

Physical therapy, especially when combined with **graded exercise** programs, is another effective method of harnessing neuroplasticity to reduce pain. Exercise has been shown to promote the release of endorphins (the body's natural painkillers) and stimulate neuroplastic changes in the brain that help retrain neural circuits involved in pain processing. Regular exercise can also reduce inflammation, improve flexibility, and increase strength, all of which contribute to the management of chronic pain.

The Future of Pain Management:Neuroplasticity as a Treatment Target

As our understanding of neuroplasticity continues to evolve, so too will the strategies for treating chronic pain. We are moving toward an era where treatments will focus not just on alleviating the symptoms of pain but also on retraining the brain to perceive pain in a healthier, more adaptive way. With the use of therapies like CBT, graded exposure, mindfulness, and targeted physical interventions, we have the potential to rewire the brain's response to pain, offering new hope for those living with chronic pain conditions.

By embracing the science of neuroplasticity, we are entering a new frontier in pain management—one where the brain's remarkable ability to change can be harnessed to create lasting relief for those who need it most.

Chapter - 4

Ethics And Challenges In Pain Management

4.1 Balancing Medication: Addiction vs. Relief

As a pain specialist, one of the most difficult and delicate challenges we face is finding the balance between providing effective pain relief and minimizing the risk of addiction to pain medications. Pain management is a critical aspect of healthcare, but it is also fraught with ethical dilemmas, particularly when it comes to the use of opioid medications. This dilemma is not just about managing the patient's pain but also about managing their long-term health, well-being, and potential risks associated with treatment.

We never take the decision to prescribe pain medication, especially opioids, lightly. Opioids can provide life-changing relief for patients experiencing severe, chronic pain. They can help individuals regain their quality of life, enabling them to perform daily activities, return to work, and restore a sense of normalcy. However, the reality is that opioid medications carry a significant risk of dependence, misuse, and, in some cases, addiction.

The Two Faces of Pain Medicine

On one hand, pain medication—especially opioids—can be a lifesaver for people suffering from acute pain after surgery, injury, or trauma, as well as for those with **chronic pain** from conditions like **cancer**, **osteoarthritis**, or **neuropathic pain**. When prescribed and managed properly, these medications can be a crucial part of a patient's recovery and pain management plan.

On the other hand, the very medications that provide relief can also create significant harm. **Opioid use disorder** (OUD) has become a widespread issue, with millions of individuals worldwide developing dependency on these drugsMisuse, higher doses than prescribed, or prolonged use of these medications increase the risk of addiction. The result can be devastating—not just for the patient's health but also for their social, emotional, and financial well-being.

The Ethical Dilemma: Providing Relief vs. Preventing Harm

As a pain specialist, I frequently find myself balancing these two perspectives: ensuring my patients receive adequate pain relief while also protecting them from the potential harms of long-term opioid use. This balancing act requires careful assessment, continuous monitoring, and a compassionate understanding of the patient's needs and concerns.

Assessing the Risk of Addiction

One of the first steps in managing pain safely is evaluating the risk of addiction for each patient. This assessment involves understanding the patient's medical history, pain levels, and mental health status. Patients with a history of substance abuse, mental health disorders, or family members with addiction problems may be at higher risk of developing a dependence on opioids.

I always make it a point to discuss openly with patients the risks associated with pain medications, explaining how addiction can develop, how to take the medication responsibly, and the importance of adhering to the prescribed dose and schedule. Education about the potential risks of addiction is crucial in empowering patients to make informed decisions about their treatment.

Strategies to Minimize Risk

To mitigate the risk of addiction, I rely on several strategies:

1. **Starting with Non-Opioid Options**: Whenever possible, I prefer to start with non-opioid pain management options, such as **NSAIDs** (non-steroidal anti-inflammatory drugs), **acetaminophen**, **muscle relaxants**, or **topical analgesics**. These can often provide sufficient relief for many patients without the risks associated with opioids.

2. **Multimodal Pain Management**: In many cases, I combine various pain relief methods, such as

physical therapy, **cognitive-behavioral therapy (CBT)**, and **relaxation techniques** like mindfulness. Multimodal approaches allow me to reduce reliance on medications while still providing effective pain management.

3. **Short-Term Use of Opioids**: When opioids are necessary, I prescribe them for the **shortest duration** possible and at the lowest effective dose. I also ensure regular follow-up appointments to monitor progress, adjust the treatment plan, and assess any signs of misuse or dependence.

4. **Using Opioid Agreements**: For patients who require opioid medication for chronic pain, I often recommend an **opioid treatment agreement**. This agreement clearly outlines expectations, including the importance of taking the medication only as prescribed, not sharing medication with others, and returning for regular check-ups. This agreement serves as a safety net for both the patient and the physician, reinforcing the collaborative nature of the pain management plan.

5. **Prescription Drug Monitoring Programs (PDMPs)**: In many regions, doctors have access to **Prescription Drug Monitoring Programs** that track patients' prescriptions for controlled substances. This tool helps identify patients who may be seeking prescriptions from multiple providers, which can be an indication of misuse.

6. **Psychosocial Support**: Chronic pain often comes with emotional and psychological challenges. I encourage patients to seek support through therapy or support groups, which can help them cope with the emotional toll of chronic pain and reduce the likelihood of turning to medication as a coping mechanism.

The Bigger Picture: The Role of the Physician in Pain Management

As a pain physician, my responsibility is not just to treat the **physical** aspects of pain but also to understand the **psychosocial** dimensions. Emotional stress, depression, anxiety, and past trauma often influence pain, making any treatment plan incomplete without addressing these underlying factors. Therefore, part of my work involves educating patients about the importance of a holistic approach to pain management—one that addresses both the **mind** and **body**.

I also have a responsibility to be an advocate for my patients, ensuring that they have access to the full range of treatments available to manage their pain safely and effectively. This includes understanding and utilizing alternative treatments such as acupuncture, chiropractic care, and medical cannabis, all of which have shown promise for certain types of pain.

But perhaps most importantly, I must remain vigilant about the evolving nature of pain management practices. The opioid crisis has taught us valuable lessons about the potential dangers of medication, but it has also sparked innovation in alternative treatments and greater emphasis on **patient-centered care**. The growing focus on **non-pharmacological** treatments, such as **neuromodulation**, **biofeedback**, and **virtual reality therapy**, represents a significant shift in how we think about and manage pain.

Conclusion: A Physician's Ethical Duty

At the end of the day, balancing the need for pain relief with the risks of medication addiction is a deeply personal and ethical decision for every pain specialist. It requires an ongoing commitment to understanding the patient as a whole—physically, emotionally, and socially—while always striving to provide the best possible care.

While the road to effective pain management is often complicated, I believe that with the right approach, we can help patients find relief while avoiding the dangers of addiction. Through careful monitoring, patient education, and a holistic treatment plan, we can navigate the delicate balance between providing relief and preventing harm.

Ultimately, my role as a pain specialist is to empower patients to take charge of their health, support them through their pain journey, and provide them with the tools they need to live their lives fully and without fear of the medications they rely on for relief.

4.2 Addressing Patients with Complex Medical Histories

As a pain specialist, one of the most challenging and rewarding aspects of my job is treating patients with complex medical histories. These individuals often come to me after having seen multiple doctors, undergone numerous tests, and tried various treatments with little success. Their cases are not straightforward, and the path to effective pain management can be uncertain. Yet, this is where my role becomes critical—not just in treating the pain itself but in understanding the complexities of each patient's overall health and crafting a personalized, multifaceted treatment plan.

The Challenge of Complex Medical Histories

When dealing with patients who have a complex medical history, there are often multiple layers to consider. These patients may have several chronic conditions that interact in unpredictable ways, making the treatment of one issue potentially aggravating another. For instance, a patient with **diabetes** and **chronic pain** may experience difficulty managing both conditions simultaneously, as medications for pain may interfere with blood sugar levels, and uncontrolled diabetes can worsen neuropathy.

Similarly, potential cardiovascular risks may limit the types of pain medications a patient with heart disease and arthritis can take.

These complexities make it essential to approach treatment in a **holistic, integrated manner**. It's not just about prescribing pain relief—it's about managing the patient's overall health, preventing complications, and minimizing any negative effects from medications.

Building a Comprehensive Treatment Plan

The first step in addressing patients with complex medical histories is a thorough and comprehensive evaluation. I take the time to understand the entirety of their medical background, including:

- **Chronic conditions** they're managing (e.g., diabetes, heart disease, obesity, etc.)
- Previous treatments they've tried and their effectiveness
- Current medications and their potential interactions
- Lifestyle factors that may affect their pain (e.g., physical activity, diet, sleep patterns, and stress levels)
- Psychological factors, including depression, anxiety, or past trauma, which may contribute to their pain perception or recovery

By adopting a holistic approach, I am able to gain a comprehensive understanding and make informed decisions about addressing each layer of the patient's condition, thereby avoiding the use of universal solutions.

Collaborative Care: Working with Other Specialists

A key element of managing complex cases is collaboration with other healthcare professionals. When treating patients with multiple medical issues, no single specialist can address all the concerns. For example, if a patient with chronic pain also suffers from severe depression or anxiety, I may recommend that they see a psychiatrist or a psychologist. Additionally, patients with comorbidities like hypertension or kidney disease may need to work closely with their primary care physician or a cardiologist or nephrologist to adjust pain medications accordingly.

Together, we closely monitor every aspect of the patient's health, ensuring that no treatment exacerbates another condition. This multidisciplinary approach allows for a broader range of therapeutic options and increases the chances of successful pain management.

Personalized Medication Management

One of the most critical elements of treating complex cases is **personalizing the treatment plan**. I may need to adjust dosages, choose medications with fewer side effects, or try alternative therapies to minimize risks. For instance:

- Non-pharmacological treatments such as physical therapy, acupuncture, biofeedback, or cognitive-behavioral therapy (CBT) might be beneficial for reducing the need for medication.
- If medication is necessary, I focus on low-dose therapies, gradually titrating doses to avoid potential adverse reactions.
- For patients with opioid dependency, I may consider a medication-assisted treatment (MAT) approach, incorporating buprenorphine or methadone as part of a long-term pain management strategy.

- For those with neuropathy, antidepressants or anticonvulsants may provide effective pain relief without the addictive risks of opioids.
- Local anesthetics, such as lidocaine patches, can be helpful for localized pain and are often a safer option for patients with cardiovascular issues.

By carefully tailoring medication to each patient's unique set of conditions, I can reduce the risks of side effects and ensure that pain relief is maximized without compromising overall health.

The Psychological Aspect of Complex Pain Management

It is essential to acknowledge the **psychological aspect** when treating patients with complex medical histories. Chronic pain doesn't just affect the body—it affects the **mind** as well. Patients often struggle with feelings of **helplessness**, **frustration**, and **depression** due to the persistent nature of their pain and the limitations their conditions place on their lives.

This emotional toll can worsen physical pain, creating a vicious cycle that becomes harder to break. As a pain specialist, I spend time building trust with my patients, encouraging them to share their emotional struggles and addressing mental health concerns alongside physical pain. I often refer patients to **mental health professionals** who specialize in chronic pain, ensuring they have the emotional support they need.

Moreover, **mind-body techniques**, such as **meditation**, **mindfulness**, and **relaxation exercises**, can help break this cycle and reduce the impact of stress and anxiety on their pain. In many cases, these techniques complement medical treatments and improve overall outcomes.

Managing Expectations and Long-Term Care

A critical aspect of managing complex patients is **setting realistic expectations**. Chronic pain can be difficult to treat, and no single approach may fully resolve it. It's important to communicate openly with patients about the goals of treatment—pain relief, improving quality of life, and enhancing functionality—rather than promising complete eradication of pain. Patients must understand that pain management is often a long-term journey and that **management strategies** may evolve over time.

Regular follow-up appointments and consistent monitoring allow me to adjust the treatment plan as necessary and keep patients informed of their progressMany patients learn to live with pain as part of their journey, and a clear, supportive path forward can significantly enhance their ability to cope.

Conclusion: Empathy and Patience in Complex Care

Treating patients with complex medical histories requires not only technical expertise but also **empathy** and **patience**. Each patient is an individual with a unique set of challenges, and effective pain management demands that I listen, understand, and work collaboratively with them to find the best path forward. Through a holistic approach, personalized treatment plans, and a multidisciplinary team, we can offer these patients the relief they deserve while ensuring that their broader health needs are met.

The process is not always easy, but it is incredibly rewarding when patients begin to experience meaningful improvements in their lives. Managing complex pain requires a careful, thoughtful approach—one that combines medical knowledge with compassion and an unwavering commitment to helping people regain their quality of life.

4.3 Dealing with Over-Diagnosis and Over-Treatment

In the realm of pain management, one of the more insidious challenges I face is the **tendency toward over-diagnosis and over-treatment.** While the aim of healthcare is undoubtedly to improve patient outcomes, there are instances where patients are subjected to unnecessary tests, treatments, or procedures that do little to alleviate their pain and may even exacerbate their condition. As a pain specialist, I am committed to finding the **balance between effective treatment** and avoiding the pitfalls of unnecessary medical intervention.

Understanding Over-Diagnosis and Over-Treatment

Over-diagnosis is the process of identifying a condition, often unnecessarily, even though it may not pose any significant harm to the patient. This is often the result of the widespread use of diagnostic technologies and tools that detect even the slightest abnormality, leading to treatments that may not be needed. Over-treatment, on the other hand, refers to medical interventions that are more aggressive or frequent than necessary for the condition at hand. In pain management, this could mean prescribing opioids without considering alternative treatments, or performing unnecessary surgeries in cases where conservative therapies would suffice.

While there are times when further investigation and interventions are indeed warranted, it is critical to recognize when these actions may be more harmful than helpful. Overdiagnosis and overtreatment can lead to a **cascade of unnecessary procedures**, which may not only add to a patient's financial burden but also increase the risk of complications and side effects and even worsen their overall condition.

The Dangers of Overdiagnosis

Overdiagnosis can be particularly problematic in pain management. Patients may undergo numerous tests and imaging studies—such as MRIs or X-rays—often revealing incidental findings that are unrelated to their symptoms. For example, a patient experiencing chronic back pain may have an MRI that shows **mild degenerative changes** in the spine, but these changes may be completely unrelated to the pain they're experiencing.

When these incidental findings are labeled as a "diagnosis," they can **lead to unnecessary anxiety**, further testing, and even treatments that may not improve the patient's quality of life. This is especially true in **musculoskeletal pain,** where aging or wear-and-tear changes may be present in imaging but may not be the actual source of pain.

It is essential to remind ourselves, ourselves and our patients, patients that **not all abnormalities in imaging studies are symptomatic**. As pain specialists, we must assess the whole person, not just what the scans reveal. Sometimes, the best approach is to avoid over-diagnosingoverdiagnosing and focus on a **thorough clinical evaluation** and the patient's reported symptoms.

The Risks of Over-TreatmentOvertreatment

Over-treatmentOvertreatment can take many forms, from **prescribing unnecessary medications** to recommending unnecessary surgeries. A significant contributor to over-treatment in pain management is the over-prescription of pain medications, especially opioids. While these medications can be incredibly effective in managing acute pain, their long-term use, particularly for chronic pain, can lead to **dependence**, **addiction**, and a host of other complications, such as **tolerance** (requiring higher doses for the same effect) and **side effects** like **constipation**, **drowsiness**, and **nausea**.

In some cases, patients are treated with opioids without exploring alternative treatments, such as **physical therapy**, **cognitive behavioral therapy (CBT)**, **acupuncture**, or **mindfulness-based stress reduction**. These non-pharmacological options can be highly effective for managing chronic pain without the risks associated with long-term medication use.

Similarly, some patients may undergo **unnecessary surgeries**. Always consider surgery as a last resort, especially when other options remain unexplored. In the case of conditions like chronic back pain or knee osteoarthritis, surgery may be proposed too early, before **physical therapy**, **lifestyle changes**, or **injections** have been fully explored.

Always consider surgery as a last resort, especially when other options remain unexplored. A patient who undergoes unnecessary treatments may begin to feel **disillusioned** with their care, leading to **increased frustration** and **distrust** in the healthcare system. This can undermine the therapeutic relationship, making it harder to engage in future treatment plans.

How I Approach Avoiding Over-Diagnosis and Over-Treatment

As a pain specialist, I am deeply committed to the principle of doing no harm first. To avoid over-diagnosisoverdiagnosis and over-treatment over-treatment, I approach every patient with an open mind and a willingness to question whether interventions are truly necessary. Here's how I navigate these issues:

1. **Thorough Evaluation and Diagnosis:** Rather than relying solely on imaging or lab tests, I conduct a comprehensive clinical evaluation. I ask detailed questions about the patient's history, lifestyle, and symptom patterns, and I perform a physical exam. This allows me to build a complete picture of the patient's condition and **rule out** issues that may be

misdiagnosed based on isolated symptoms or test results.

2. **Conservative Treatment First:** I typically start with **conservative treatments**, such as physical therapy, exercise, **cognitive behavioral therapy**, or lifestyle adjustments, before moving on to more invasive options like injections or surgery. Many patients find relief through these less aggressive approaches, and it's always my goal to minimize the need for heavy medications or surgical intervention.

3. **Shared Decision-Making:** I believe in working **collaboratively** with my patients. I take the time to explain my reasoning behind each treatment recommendation and offer a range of options when possible. This allows patients to make informed decisions about their care, and it also encourages them to be active participants in their treatment journey.

4. **Regular Monitoring and Adjustments:** I regularly assess the effectiveness of treatment plans and adjust them as necessary. If a treatment isn't working, we move on to the next step, but I always try to avoid escalating care too quickly. For example, if a patient isn't responding to oral medications, I may suggest exploring options like **topical treatments**, **nerve blocks**, or **physical therapy** before resorting to more potent drugs.

5. **Avoiding Overuse of Diagnostic Tests:** Diagnostic tests are important tools, but I am cautious about over-relying on them, particularly when imaging

studies are concerned. I focus on clinical findings and listen closely to what the patient is telling me. In many cases, these clinical insights are far more important than any scan.

Conclusion: The Importance of Thoughtful, Ethical Care

Over-diagnosis Overdiagnosis and overtreatment overtreatment are not just professional pitfalls—they are deeply personal. Unnecessary tests, medications, and procedures often cause patients to experience greater distress, confusion, and frustration. As a pain specialist, my priority is to practice thoughtful, ethical care that prioritizes the patient's well-being over convenience or the desire for quick fixes.

By sticking to a patient-centered approach, focusing on evidence-based treatments, and avoiding unnecessary interventions, we can help our patients achieve meaningful pain relief while minimizing harm. Ultimately, the goal is not to treat the, diagnosis but to treat the **person**—with compassion, integrity, and respect for their individual needs and circumstances.

4.4 Advocating for Non-Surgical Solutions in a Surgical World

Advocating for non-surgical alternatives in a healthcare environment where surgical interventions are often perceived as the ultimate solution to pain can be challenging. Yet, as a pain specialist, I believe it is my responsibility to advocate for **non-surgical solutions** whenever possible. While surgery may be necessary in certain situations, it should never be the first or automatic option. In a world where we often turn to the operating room as the solution to our problems, it is critical to remember that **surgery is not always the answer**—and it comes with significant risks.

The Surgical Bias in Modern Medicine

In many medical fields, surgery is still viewed as the most definitive and "authoritative" solution to a problem. The medical community has placed a high value on the tangible, immediate results that surgeries can provide. This bias has been perpetuated by medical advancements, the marketing power of surgical specialties, and a public perception that surgery equals a "quick fix" to chronic issues.

For pain management, especially in cases of musculoskeletal pain like **chronic back pain**, **knee osteoarthritis**, or **spinal disc herniation**, surgery is often presented as the go-to treatment option. Surgeons, understandably, are trained to intervene surgically; in some cases, surgery is indeed the most effective course of action. However, surgery comes with risks, both immediate (such as infection, anesthesia complications, and surgical errors) and long-term (including the potential for **post-surgical pain**, **scar tissue formation**, and **failed back surgery syndrome**).

What many patients—and even some doctors—don't realize is that **non-surgical solutions** can be just as effective, if not more so, for managing chronic pain and improving quality of life. As someone who works closely with patients seeking alternatives to surgery, it is my goal to provide **education** and **guidance** on the full range of treatment options available. The key lies in identifying the root cause of pain, understanding the patient's lifestyle, and choosing the least invasive option that will provide the most sustainable relief.

Why Non-Surgical Options Should Be Considered First

Non-surgical treatments for pain are often less invasive, less costly, and come with far fewer risks than surgery. In many cases, the benefits of non-surgical interventions far outweigh the risks, especially for individuals suffering from chronic pain conditions. Here's why I advocate for non-surgical solutions:

1. **Fewer Risks**: Surgery, by its very nature, introduces risk. Every time a patient undergoes anesthesia or a surgical procedure, there is the potential for complications, including infection, bleeding, or damage to surrounding tissue. Non-surgical treatments, such as **physical therapy**, **injections**, or **acupuncture**, have significantly fewer risks and are often just as effective in managing pain.

2. **Long-Term Sustainability**: Surgery may provide immediate relief, but it doesn't always address the underlying issues that caused the pain in the first place. Non-surgical treatments, on the other hand, aim to **strengthen the body**, **improve mobility**, and **restore function**, which can lead to longer-lasting results. For example, physical therapy focuses on improving strength, flexibility, and posture, all of which can reduce the likelihood of pain returning.

3. **Cost-Effectiveness**: Surgery is often a costly procedure, especially when factoring in hospital stays, post-surgery care, rehabilitation, and lost wages due to time off work. Non-surgical treatments tend to be more affordable and accessible, especially when coupled with preventative measures that can reduce the need for more drastic interventions.

4. **Holistic Approach**: Non-surgical treatments often take a more **holistic approach** to pain management. They not only aim to reduce pain, but they also focus on improving overall well-being. This might include **lifestyle changes**, **nutrition advice**, **stress reduction techniques**, or even **mind-body therapies**. Addressing pain in this way can lead to broader improvements in the patient's quality of life, rather than just focusing on the immediate issue.

5. **Faster Recovery**: The recovery time for non-surgical treatments is typically far quicker than for surgery. While recovery from a major surgery can take weeks or even months, many non-surgical treatments, such as **physical therapy** or **cortisone injections**, can offer relief within a matter of days to weeks, allowing patients to return to their normal lives more quickly.

Non-Surgical SolutionsSolutions : A Closer Look

Here are some of the non-surgical options that I frequently recommend to my patients:

1. **Physical Therapy**: Tailored exercise programs can help to restore strength, flexibility, and proper alignment, reducing the need for surgical

intervention. Physical therapists use a combination of exercises, manual therapy, and modalities like heat or cold therapy to treat musculoskeletal pain effectively.

2. **Pain Injections**: For conditions like **joint pain** or **nerve-related pain**, injections such as **steroid injections**, **nerve blocks**, or **hyaluronic acid injections** can provide significant relief. These injections are minimally invasive, offer targeted pain relief, and allow the patient to avoid the risks and recovery time associated with surgery.

3. **Regenerative Medicine**: The use of **stem cells**, **platelet-rich plasma (PRP)**, or **prolotherapy** is growing as an alternative to surgery. These treatments focus on stimulating the body's own healing process, reducing inflammation, and regenerating damaged tissues. While still evolving, regenerative medicine is showing promising results for conditions like **osteoarthritis** and **tendon injuries**.

4. **Lifestyle Modifications**: Simple changes in daily habits can have a huge impact on pain management. For instance, improving posture, maintaining a healthy weight, or adjusting ergonomic setups at work can help reduce the strain on the body and prevent chronic pain from worsening.

5. **Cognitive Behavioral Therapy (CBT)**: For many patients, **psychological factors** play a significant role in pain perception. CBT is a highly effective tool for managing chronic pain, as it helps patients

change the way they think about and respond to their pain. Through this approach, patients can develop coping strategies that improve their ability to handle pain without relying on medications or surgery.

6. **Mindfulness and Meditation**: **Mindfulness-based practices** have been shown to reduce pain perception and improve emotional resilience in the face of chronic pain. These techniques help patients relax, manage stress, and gain better control over their body's pain responses.

The Role of the Pain Specialist in Advocacy

Being a patient advocate is crucial to my job as a pain specialist. I prioritize educating my patients about all available treatment options, instead of relying solely on surgery as the initial course of action. While surgery may sometimes be necessary, it is my duty to explore **conservative options first** and only recommend surgical intervention if absolutely necessary.

I also aim to create an **open dialogue** with my patients, empowering them to make informed decisions about their care. By elucidating the advantages and disadvantages of each treatment option, offering evidence-based recommendations, and guiding them through the decision-making process, I aim to steer my patients towards the optimal outcome, be it avoiding surgery or opting for it as a final resort.

Conclusion: Rethinking Pain Treatment

Surgery is not always the panacea we hope for. In fact, non-surgical solutions often provide more sustainable, cost-effective, and low-risk relief for patients. By advocating for non-surgical treatments and empowering patients to explore a range of options, we can help them not only manage their pain more effectively but also improve their overall health and well-being.

As we move forward, I hope that more patients and healthcare professionals begin to view non-surgical pain management as a **first-line option**, option rather than an afterthought. Ultimately, my aim is to establish a healthcare environment that prioritizes holistic, thoughtful, and patient-centered care, acknowledging surgery as merely one component of a broader picture.

4.5 The Emotional Cost of Chronic Pain

Chronic pain doesn’t just affect the body—it seeps into the mind, the heart, and the spirit. For those living with persistent, long-term pain, the emotional toll can be as profound and debilitating as the physical symptoms themselves. Chronic pain is a complex experience that can trigger a range of emotions, from frustration and sadness to hopelessness and isolation. As a pain specialist, I’ve seen firsthand how **the emotional cost of chronic pain** can often overshadow the physical pain, leaving patients feeling trapped and overwhelmed.

Understanding the Emotional Impact

Living with chronic pain is a constant challenge that shapes a person's daily life. The **emotional toll** often begins long before the first signs of physical discomfort. Over time, the continuous struggle with pain can lead to emotional exhaustion. Patients may feel like they are on a never-ending roller coaster, caught in cycles of relief followed by relapse, which erodes their sense of hope and well-being.

The emotional impact of chronic pain can manifest in several ways:

1. **Depression:** It's not uncommon for those suffering from chronic pain to develop depression. In fact, studies have shown that people with chronic pain are significantly more likely to experience clinical **depression** than the general population. The constant battle with pain, the inability to perform daily tasks, and the frustration of failed treatments can make a person feel helpless and emotionally drained. This can spiral into feelings of **worthlessness**, **loss of interest in activities**, and a general sense of despair.

2. **Anxiety**: The unpredictability of chronic pain can also lead to **anxiety**. Pain is often exacerbated by stress, and the fear of future flare-ups can become overwhelming. Patients may constantly worry about the next episode of pain, its intensity, or whether they will be able to manage it. The emotional stress that comes with this anxiety can heighten the perception of pain, creating a vicious cycle that's difficult to break.

3. **Anger and Frustration**: Chronic pain can also stir up anger and frustration, especially when it feels like no one truly understands what the patient is going through. This can lead to feelings of **resentment**, both toward the condition and the people around

them. Patients may feel misunderstood by family, friends, or even healthcare providers, which compounds their sense of isolation.

4. **Guilt and Shame**: Many individuals with chronic pain experience **guilt** or **shame** for not being able to keep up with their usual responsibilities. Whether it's caring for children, going to work, or maintaining social relationships, the limitations imposed by pain can make individuals feel inadequate or like a burden to others. This emotional weight can severely impact self-esteem, leading to withdrawal from social interactions and feelings of isolation.

5. **Isolation**: Over time, the physical limitations of chronic pain can force individuals to withdraw from their social circles, leading to a profound sense of **loneliness**. They may avoid social gatherings or activities they once enjoyed, either because they don't have the energy or because they fear their pain will be visible. The result is an emotional isolation that can deepen the already-present feelings of depression and anxiety.

6. **Grief and Loss**: Chronic pain often forces individuals to grieve the loss of their previous life. The person they once were—the one who could walk, run, work, or play without pain—feels like a distant memory. This sense of loss can be deeply mournful, as they come to terms with the limitations imposed by their condition. It's important to understand that grief over one's health and

capabilities is a valid, natural response to chronic pain.

The Interconnectedness of Body and Mind

What many people don't fully realize is how intertwined physical pain and emotional pain truly are. The mind-body connection plays a crucial role in the experience of pain. Chronic pain can change the brain's neurochemistry, increasing sensitivity to pain and altering mood. This can lead to the development of chronic pain syndrome, where emotional distress worsens the perception of pain and vice versa.

For example, when patients experience emotional stress, their muscles tense, and their bodies become more sensitive to pain. In turn, the increased pain leads to more emotional distress, creating a feedback loop that intensifies the overall experience. Conversely, the emotional distress caused by pain can reduce a person's ability to cope with the discomfort, making it feel even worse. Understanding the mind-body connection is essential in addressing the emotional cost of chronic pain. A holistic approach that includes both physical and emotional healing is often the most effective way to break this cycle.

Approaching the Emotional Aspects of Pain Management

As a pain specialist, it's critical to address not just the physical symptoms of chronic pain, pain but also the **emotional and psychological impacts** it has on my patients. Often, a combination of physical treatments and emotional support is necessary to create a comprehensive pain management plan. Here are a few approaches that can help:

1. **Psychological Support**: Counseling or therapy can play a vital role in managing the emotional cost of chronic pain. **Cognitive-behavioral therapy (CBT)**, for instance, is a proven approach that helps patients recognize and change negative thought patterns associated with pain. It can help individuals **reframe their perception of pain**, develop **coping strategies**, and **reduce emotional distress**.

2. **Mindfulness and Relaxation Techniques**: Practices like **mindfulness meditation**, **deep breathing**, and **guided imagery** can help reduce the emotional strain of chronic pain. These techniques teach patients how to **relax their minds** and bodies, leading to a reduction in pain perception and stress. Mindfulness, in particular, encourages individuals to live in the present moment, helping to break the cycle of anxiety about the future and regret over the past.

3. **Support Groups**: Joining a **support group** where others share similar experiences can be incredibly empowering. Chronic pain patients often feel isolated, but connecting with others who understand their struggles can help them feel less alone. Emotional support from peers can provide comfort, understanding, and validation of their pain, which is vital for emotional healing.

4. **Self-Care**: Encouraging self-care practices is another important aspect of managing the emotional toll of chronic pain. Taking time to engage in activities that bring joy or relaxation—whether that's reading, painting, gardening, or simply enjoying nature—can provide a much-needed emotional escape from the constant battle with pain.
5. **Education**: Educating patients about the mind-body connection and the emotional aspects of pain is essential. When patients understand that their emotional experiences are a valid and natural part of the pain journey, they may be less likely to internalize feelings of guilt or shame. Instead, they can begin to embrace **healing on both levels**, recognizing that emotional care is just as important as physical care.

Conclusion: Healing the Whole Person

Chronic pain is not just a physical challenge; it's an emotional journey that requires compassion, understanding, and care. As a pain specialist, I strive to offer my patients not only the most effective physical treatments but also the emotional support they need to navigate the complex terrain of chronic pain. By acknowledging the **emotional cost** of living with chronic pain, we can move beyond simply managing symptoms and begin to help our patients heal as a whole person—body, mind, and spirit.

Pain may be inevitable, but **suffering is optional**. With the right tools, support, and a comprehensive approach to healing, chronic pain does not have to define a person's life. With the right mindset, treatment, and compassion, we can transform the emotional journey of chronic pain. Through a holistic approach, we can give patients the opportunity to reclaim their **emotional health** and **quality of life** alongside the physical relief they so desperately need.

Chapter - 5

Building Collaborative Healthcare

5.1 Working with Physiotherapists and Nutritionists

Effective pain management extends far beyond the clinic, involving an integrated approach that brings together a multidisciplinary team of healthcare professionals. As a pain specialist, I've witnessed the profound benefits of working closely with physiotherapists and nutritionists. Together, we form a comprehensive support system that helps patients manage pain more effectively, not just by treating symptoms but by addressing the root causes. It's a powerful, collaborative effort that ultimately enhances the patient's well-being.

The Role of Physiotherapists in Pain Management

Physiotherapists play a critical role in helping patients recover from injury, manage chronic conditions, and restore movement. When a person is living with chronic pain, especially from musculoskeletal disorders like **arthritis** or **back pain**, the **physical component** of pain management becomes essential. Physiotherapists are trained to assess and treat the musculoskeletal system through hands-on techniques, exercise prescription, and education, making them indispensable in the care of patients with pain.

Physiotherapy isn't just about alleviating pain—it's about teaching patients to **move correctly**, **build strength**, and **maintain mobility**. For patients suffering from chronic pain, the right exercises can help improve posture, flexibility, and strength, reducing the pressure on painful areas and enabling the body to function more efficiently. Here are some ways in which physiotherapists assist in pain management:

1. **Movement Re-education**: Physiotherapists teach patients how to move correctly, using postural training and body mechanics techniques to reduce strain on the body. Proper movement patterns can make a significant difference in preventing pain flare-ups and improving long-term outcomes.

2. **Strengthening Exercises**: Targeted strengthening exercises help restore function and reduce the impact of chronic pain. By strengthening the muscles around a painful joint or body part, physiotherapists can alleviate pressure on the affected area, promoting better alignment and support.

3. **Manual Therapy**: Techniques such as **massage**, **joint mobilizations**, and **stretching** help release tension, increase circulation, and promote flexibility. These interventions can reduce stiffness and improve

mobility, particularly for patients with conditions like arthritis or muscular tension.

4. **Pain Education**: Physiotherapists also play a vital role in educating patients about their condition. They teach patients about the **nature of their pain**, how movement and posture can influence pain levels, and how to avoid behaviors that may exacerbate symptoms.

5. **Gradual Return to Activity**: For individuals who have been living with pain for some time, the idea of returning to normal activities can feel daunting. Physiotherapists guide patients through the process, helping them gradually reintroduce activity in a safe and controlled manner, which can significantly reduce the risk of injury and re-injury.

The Role of Nutritionists in Pain Management

Nutrition is often an overlooked aspect of pain management, but it plays a pivotal role in the overall health and well-being of patients dealing with chronic pain. The foods we eat can have a direct impact on inflammation, pain perception, and healing processes. As a pain specialist, I often collaborate with **nutritionists** to help patients adopt dietary habits that support their pain management goals.

A proper diet can reduce inflammation, support tissue repair, and even alleviate the severity of certain pain conditions. Nutritionists can provide patients with specific dietary strategies to manage their pain, improve their energy levels, and optimize their overall health.

Here are some ways nutritionists contribute to pain management:

1. **Anti-Inflammatory Diet**: Chronic inflammation is a key factor in many pain conditions, such as **rheumatoid arthritis**, **osteoarthritis**, and **fibromyalgia**. Nutritionists can recommend an **anti-inflammatory diet**, rich in foods like **fruits**, **vegetables**, **whole grains**, **lean proteins**, and **healthy fats** (e.g., omega-3 fatty acids from fish and flaxseeds). These foods help reduce the body's inflammatory response, providing relief from pain and improving overall health.
2. **Weight Management**: For patients dealing with **joint pain**, particularly in areas like the knees and hips, managing weight is crucial. Extra weight places additional stress on the joints, exacerbating pain and potentially leading to further damage. Nutritionists play an essential role in helping patients achieve and maintain a healthy weight by advising on portion control, calorie intake, and making healthier food choices.
3. **Managing Food Sensitivities and Allergies**: Some patients may have food sensitivities or allergies that contribute to inflammation and pain. A nutritionist can help identify trigger foods—such as gluten, dairy, or certain processed foods—that may be exacerbating pain symptoms. By adjusting their diet, patients can see an improvement in their pain levels and overall health.

4. **Micronutrients for Pain Relief**: Certain vitamins and minerals, such as **Vitamin D**, **magnesium**, **curcumin** (found in turmeric), and **ginger**, have anti-inflammatory and pain-relieving properties. Nutritionists can guide patients in incorporating these micronutrients into their diet through food sources or supplements to support pain relief and healing.

5. **Hydration**: Staying hydrated is essential for overall health, and dehydration can worsen certain types of pain, particularly muscle and joint pain. Nutritionists emphasize the importance of proper hydration and can guide patients on how much water to consume daily based on their individual needs.

Collaboration for Holistic Pain Management

One of the most significant advantages of collaborating with physiotherapists and nutritionists is the ability to provide **holistic care**. A variety of factors, including physical fitness, nutritional habits, and mental health, influence pain, which doesn't exist in isolation. By working together, we can develop a comprehensive treatment plan that addresses all aspects of a patient's life, giving them the best chance for long-term relief.

Here's how this collaboration benefits patients:

1. **Comprehensive Care**: Each healthcare professional brings a unique skill set to the table, allowing for a well-rounded approach to pain management. As a pain specialist, I focus on identifying the underlying cause of pain and recommending appropriate treatments. Physiotherapists help patients restore

physical function, while nutritionists work on improving the body's internal environment through diet. Together, we ensure that all aspects of the patient's health are considered.

2. **Patient-Centered Treatment**: A collaborative approach allows us to customize treatment plans based on the patient's specific needs. Whether a patient requires a more intensive physiotherapy regimen or specific dietary changes, we can tailor our approach to suit their lifestyle, preferences, and health goals.

3. **Increased Motivation and Support**: Patients often feel more empowered when they have a team of professionals supporting them. The collaboration between physiotherapists, nutritionists, and pain specialists provides a **supportive network** that helps patients stay motivated and engaged in their recovery process. This increased level of support can make a significant difference in a patient's ability to manage pain and adopt healthier habits.

4. **Better Outcomes**: Studies show that patients who receive multidisciplinary care often experience better outcomes than those who receive treatment from a single provider. By addressing pain from multiple angles—physical, nutritional, and emotional—we can achieve more comprehensive, long-lasting results.

Conclusion: The Power of Teamwork

Managing chronic pain requires a team approach—one that acknowledges the complexity of pain and addresses it from all angles. Physiotherapists and nutritionists are crucial members of the healthcare team, providing specialized care that complements the work of pain specialists. By collaborating with these professionals, we can offer patients a holistic and personalized treatment plan that not only alleviates pain but also promotes healing, overall health, and long-term wellness.

Through this collaborative approach, patients have the opportunity to reclaim control over their pain, restore their physical and emotional well-being, and live a more active, fulfilling life. Together, we can create a supportive, healing environment that truly makes a difference in the lives of those living with pain.

5.2 The Role of Family Support in Pain Recovery

Pain doesn't just affect the person experiencing it; it touches the lives of everyone around them. Family plays an often underestimated but crucial role in the **recovery process** for individuals suffering from chronic pain. As a pain specialist, I've witnessed firsthand how family members can either enhance or hinder the healing journey. In many cases, their support—emotionally, physically, and mentally—can be the difference between long-term pain management and long-term suffering.

The Emotional Impact of Chronic Pain on Families

Chronic pain is a deeply emotional experience for both the individual suffering from it and their loved ones. Over time, living with persistent pain can lead to feelings of frustration, helplessness, and sadness for both parties. For the person in pain, it often means dealing with feelings of isolation, depression, and anxiety about their future. For family members, watching a loved one struggle without being able to "fix" the problem can create feelings of **guilt**, **stress**, and **fatigue**.

Family support is essential not just for providing comfort but for helping the individual with chronic pain feel **validated** in their experiences. Many patients with chronic pain feel misunderstood, especially when their pain is invisible or not immediately apparent to others. Family members who are empathetic and well-informed can provide emotional validation, helping to reduce feelings of isolation.

In the recovery journey, family members often serve as the **emotional anchor**. When they actively listen, offer encouragement, and acknowledge the emotional toll of chronic pain, they help create a healing environment. This emotional connection can directly influence the patient's ability to cope with pain, adhere to treatment plans, and ultimately experience relief.

Practical Support: Creating a Pain-Friendly Home Environment

Pain recovery doesn't just happen in a doctor's office or during physical therapy sessions; it's an ongoing process that takes place in the home. One of the most important ways that family members can assist is by helping to create a **pain-friendly environment**.

This involves several practical steps that make life easier for the person in pain:

1. **Managing Daily Tasks**: Chronic pain often makes routine activities, such as cleaning, cooking, or even bathing, a significant challenge. Family members can step in to help with these tasks, reducing the burden on the person suffering from pain. Whether it's helping with meal prep or assisting with mobility, these gestures go a long way in improving the individual's quality of life.
2. **Creating a Comfortable Space**: A calm and comfortable living space can make a huge difference in managing pain. Family members can help adjust the home environment to ensure it is **ergonomically friendly**, using supportive furniture, reducing clutter, and ensuring proper lighting to make movement easier. A peaceful, clutter-free environment can help reduce stress levels, which in turn can help reduce pain intensity.
3. **Encouraging Movement and Exercise**: Encouraging light movement and exercise—whether it's going for a short walk or participating in stretching exercises—can be a challenge for someone in chronic pain. However, family members who encourage and even participate in these activities can create a **motivating environment** that encourages physical rehabilitation. Whether it's joining in for a walk or helping the person get to physical therapy, this support can make a significant impact on recovery.
4. **Accompanying Medical Appointments**: Attending medical appointments together shows the person

suffering from chronic pain that they're not alone in their recovery. Family members can act as advocates, helping the patient remember important questions or information, and offering moral support during treatments or therapies.

Communication: The Bridge Between the Patient and Their Family

Effective communication is perhaps one of the most powerful tools in the pain recovery process. When family members are well-informed about the nature of the pain and treatment options, they are better equipped to offer the **right kind of support**. Communication can include discussing the patient's **treatment plans**, **symptoms**, and **challenges** with the healthcare team. By actively participating in these conversations, family members become allies in the healing process.

But beyond the logistics of treatment, open communication also means creating a **space for the patient to express themselves emotionally**. Chronic pain often comes with feelings of **guilt**, **fear**, and **frustration**—all of which need to be expressed for healing to occur. Families can offer a supportive listening ear without judgment, allowing the individual in pain to feel heard and understood. This creates a deeper sense of emotional intimacy and trust, which can significantly enhance recovery.

Moreover, good communication helps establish realistic expectations. Both the patient and family members need to understand that recovery from chronic pain is often a gradual process. It involves setbacks, difficult days, and small victories. By having open conversations about what the patient is experiencing, families can adjust their expectations, manage frustrations, and maintain a more balanced approach to the recovery journey.

Family Dynamics: Challenges and Adjustments

While family support is essential, it's important to acknowledge that chronic pain can create strains within family relationships. The roles and dynamics within the household may shift, with family members taking on additional caregiving duties. For some, this can lead to **caregiver burnout**, resentment, or strained relationships. It's important for family members to recognize their own **emotional and physical limits**. Seeking support from counselors, support groups, or even taking breaks when needed is key to avoiding burnout and maintaining a healthy family dynamic.

Additionally, some family members may struggle with **understanding** the extent of the pain, especially if it is invisible. This lack of understanding can lead to **frustration** or **impatience**. In these cases, open, honest conversations and education about the nature of chronic pain—what it feels like, how it impacts day-to-day life, and how it fluctuates—can help everyone in the family become more empathetic and supportive.

The Ripple Effect: How Family Support Fuels Recovery

The influence of family support extends beyond just making daily life more manageable. It fuels the recovery process in more profound ways. Research shows that individuals who feel **emotionally supported** and **cared for** by family members experience **better pain outcomes**, better adherence to treatment plans, and improved mental health. Positive family relationships can reduce stress levels, which is crucial since **stress exacerbates pain**.

Furthermore, a family who is actively involved in the pain management process encourages the patient to stay **committed to their recovery plan**. Whether it's sticking to physical therapy schedules, maintaining a healthy diet, or practicing relaxation techniques, family involvement ensures that the person in pain has both the practical and emotional tools to succeed in their healing journey.

Conclusion: The Strength of Family in Healing

The recovery from chronic pain is a shared journey. Healthcare professionals often assume responsibility for pain management, but it's evident that family support holds equaL importance. Family members provide **emotional reassurance**, **practical assistance**, and **motivational support** that is indispensable for effective pain management. Their involvement fosters a healing environment that encourages recovery not just physically, physically but emotionally and mentally as well.

The journey toward healing from chronic pain is not one that should be undertaken alone. With a supportive family by their side, patients are better equipped to face the challenges of chronic pain, increase their quality of life, and find hope in their recovery process.

5.3 Collaborations with Mental Health Professionals

The connection between **mental health** and **chronic pain** is undeniable, and it is often this intersection that forms the crux of successful pain management. As a pain specialist, I cannot overstate the importance of collaborating with mental health professionals in the treatment of chronic pain. The mind and body are inextricably linked, and an integrated, holistic approach that addresses both the emotional and physical aspects of pain is essential for true healing.

Chronic pain can be emotionally and psychologically draining, and it is not uncommon for those experiencing it to develop co-existing mental health conditions such as **anxiety**, **depression**, or **post-traumatic stress disorder (PTSD)**. These conditions not only affect a person's emotional well-being but can also **exacerbate pain** symptoms, creating a vicious cycle that's difficult to break. On the other hand, the mental health of individuals can be **neglected** when chronic pain is the primary focus of care. This is where collaboration with mental health professionals becomes crucial.

The Impact of Mental Health on Pain Perception

When a patient suffers from chronic pain, it is not just the physical sensation that is affecting them. Pain is multidimensional, impacting mood, behavior, and overall mental well-being. Research shows that emotional stress and negative psychological states can worsen the perception of pain, amplifying its intensity and duration. Conditions like anxiety and depression are known to lower pain thresholds, meaning individuals are likely to experience pain as more severe and more frequent than they otherwise might.

Furthermore, chronic pain often leads to a sense of helplessness and **loss of control**, which can spiral into feelings of **hopelessness**. This creates a mental state that is **counterproductive** to healing. When individuals feel emotionally drained or trapped in the cycle of pain, it can be difficult for them to engage in treatment, follow through on prescribed exercises, or remain motivated to work toward recovery.

This is where mental health professionals' expertise comes into play. They can help **address the emotional toll** of chronic pain by **managing stress**, **reducing anxiety**, and **providing coping strategies**. Incorporating therapies such as **cognitive-behavioral therapy (CBT)**, **mindfulness practices**, or **relaxation techniques** can help patients better manage their pain, both physically and emotionally.

Integrated Pain Management: A Collaborative Approach

The collaboration between pain specialists and mental health professionals is an essential aspect of **integrated pain management**. A team-based approach provides both physical and psychological care simultaneously to create a comprehensive treatment plan.

Mental health professionals such as psychologists, psychiatrists, and counselors work alongside pain specialists to:

1. **Assess Emotional Well-Being**: Mental health professionals are trained to assess the emotional and psychological aspects of a patient's condition. By identifying mental health concerns, they can provide an accurate assessment of how these issues might be affecting the patient's pain experience.

2. **Provide Psychological Support**: Chronic pain often causes emotional distress. Professionals in mental health can provide emotional support, helping patients to cope with feelings of frustration, anxiety, and depression. This support gives patients the tools to not only manage their emotional struggles but also to stay engaged in their recovery process.

3. **Offer Pain-Coping Strategies**: Mental health professionals introduce patients to various coping strategies that can help them manage pain. **Cognitive-behavioral therapy (CBT)**, for example, helps patients reframe negative thought patterns that increase pain perception and emotional distress. Patients learn how to view pain differently, allowing them to feel more in control of their experience.

4. **Improve Self-Efficacy**: Self-efficacy, or the belief that one can manage their own health, is a vital factor in recovery. Mental health professionals help patients build self-efficacy through various therapeutic techniques, helping them regain the sense of control that pain often takes away.

5. **Support Behavioral Changes**: Mental health professionals are skilled in helping patients make behavior changes that can improve both their mental

and physical health. Whether it's **improving sleep habits**, **engaging in physical activity**, or **adhering to treatment plans**, these changes contribute to pain management.

Specific Therapies in Pain Management

The most effective collaboration between mental health professionals and pain specialists is often achieved through **specific therapeutic interventions** tailored to the patient's unique needs. These therapies go beyond traditional medication and physical treatments to address the **psychological components** of chronic pain.

- **Cognitive-Behavioral Therapy (CBT)**: One of the most widely used therapies in managing chronic pain, CBT helps patients identify and alter negative thoughts and behaviors that intensify their pain experience. By focusing on **thought patterns**, CBT empowers patients to shift their mindset, improving their perception of pain and their ability to manage it.
- **Mindfulness-Based Stress Reduction (MBSR)**: Mindfulness techniques, such as meditation and deep-breathing exercises, have been shown to reduce pain perception and enhance coping mechanisms. By practicing mindfulness, individuals learn to become more aware of their pain without becoming overwhelmed by it.
- **Biofeedback**: This technique teaches individuals to control bodily functions, such as heart rate and muscle tension, which can impact pain levels.

Biofeedback can help patients reduce stress and anxiety that often accompany chronic pain.

- **Acceptance and Commitment Therapy (ACT)**: ACT focuses on helping patients accept their pain, rather than trying to avoid it, and commit to living a meaningful life despite it. It helps patients develop resilience and the ability to continue functioning well even in the face of pain.

Breaking the Stigma: A Holistic View of Pain

Integrating mental health care into pain management also helps reduce the stigma that often surrounds chronic pain, particularly its psychosomatic nature.

Many patients suffering from chronic pain feel as though their pain is not taken seriously, especially when it is linked to mental health conditions such as depression or anxiety.

This stigma can discourage individuals from seeking help, leaving them to suffer in silence. However, the growing understanding of the interplay between mental health and pain challenges the notion that chronic pain is solely physical. By acknowledging the psychological aspects of pain and working collaboratively with mental health professionals, we foster an environment where **holistic** care becomes the standard, not the exception.

Conclusion: A Unified Approach to Healing

In the world of chronic pain management, a collaborative approach between pain specialists and mental health professionals is not just recommended; it is essential. Pain does not exist in isolation from the mind; it affects the body, mind, and emotions in complex ways. By combining expertise in both pain management and mental health care, we offer patients the best possible chance at healing—physically, mentally, and emotionally.

As healthcare professionals, we must recognize that pain management extends beyond prescribing medications or performing procedures. True healing happens when we treat the whole person, not just the symptoms. Only through collaboration can we offer patients the comprehensive care they deserve, empowering them to regain control over their pain and their lives.

5.4 Referrals and Second Opinions: Ensuring the Best Outcome

In the field of pain management, no one specialist can possess all the answers, nor should they. Pain is complex, and each individual's experience is unique. There will be times when a patient's needs extend beyond what I can provide, and when that happens, the most responsible thing I can do is **refer** them to another expert who can offer the specialized care they need. It is my belief that referrals and second opinions are not signs of failure—they are an essential part of providing the **best possible care**.

Chronic pain can be overwhelming, and navigating the healthcare system can sometimes feel like an insurmountable task. As a pain specialist, my job is to not only diagnose and treat pain but to also ensure that my patients are receiving the most comprehensive and holistic care available. This includes knowing when to call on colleagues from other specialties or encourage a second opinion when necessary.

Why Referrals Matter

Referrals are about finding the right fit for the patient's needs. For example, a person struggling with chronic back pain may initially visit a pain management clinic like mine. However, after a thorough assessment, I might recognize that their condition requires the attention of a **neurologist**, **orthopedic surgeon**, or **physical therapist**—experts in areas beyond my specialization. In such cases, the most effective course of action is to refer them to someone who can offer a different perspective, more advanced technology, or specialized expertise.

Referrals also extend beyond specialists; they can also involve coordinating with other healthcare providers, like **nutritionists**, **mental health professionals**, or **rehabilitation therapists**, who can contribute significantly to pain relief and management.

By making the right referrals, we ensure that patients have access to the **full spectrum** of care, which is often the key to achieving lasting relief.

The Power of a Second Opinion

Sometimes, patients may feel uncertain or uncomfortable with their treatment plan, especially if the pain persists despite ongoing care. It's natural to question whether the treatment being provided is the best approach, and a second opinion can provide peace of mind, offer a new perspective, or even suggest an entirely different treatment path.

For me, providing a second opinion is not about challenging my expertise; it's about giving the patient **confidence** that they are making the most informed decisions about their health. It also ensures that they are **not missing any potential treatment options**. Pain management is an evolving field, and new therapies, treatments, and technologies emerge all the time. A second opinion allows the patient to stay current with the latest advancements in care.

Moreover, a second opinion can **validate** the treatment plan already in place, reassuring the patient that they are on the right track. In certain instances, it could clarify the necessity for further tests or interventions. Seeking a second opinion is not about doubt, but about ensuring comprehensive care for the patient.

When to Recommend Referrals or Second Opinions

While every patient is unique, there are common scenarios where referrals and second opinions can make a significant difference in the treatment process:

1. **Persistent or Unexplained Pain**: If a patient's pain continues despite treatment, or if the source of the pain remains unclear, it may be time to seek the expertise of a specialist who can provide a fresh perspective or advanced diagnostic tools.
2. **Complex Medical Histories**: When a patient has multiple underlying health conditions that may be

contributing to their pain, it's essential to bring in specialists who can address those specific areas. For instance, a patient with both **autoimmune disorders** and chronic pain may benefit from a **rheumatologist** alongside their pain management provider.

3. **Surgical Considerations**: Sometimes, the path to healing may involve surgical intervention, but that decision should not be taken lightly. If surgery is being considered, a second opinion from a **surgeon** or a **pain management expert** who specializes in non-invasive treatments might be necessary to ensure that the most effective approach is being taken.

4. **Psychosocial Factors**: Pain is not just physical—mental health plays a huge role. If the patient's pain seems to be compounded by psychological stress, depression, or anxiety, a referral to a **psychologist** or **psychiatrist** can be invaluable. Their expertise in **cognitive-behavioral therapy (CBT)** or other mental health approaches can offer patients the tools they need to manage both the mental and physical aspects of pain.

5. **Need for Advanced Pain Management**: If pain relief is proving difficult to achieve through standard methods, it might be time to refer to a pain clinic with advanced techniques such as **nerve blocks**, **epidural injections**, or **neuromodulation therapy**. These specialized treatments often require a team of pain specialists to work together to design the most effective course of action.

Navigating the Referral Process

Referrals to other doctors can feel like a setback or a failure for many patients. They may perceive a delay in their journey or a feeling of being shuffled around unnecessarily.

As a pain specialist, I understand this concern and make every effort to explain why the referral is necessary and beneficial. I always ensure that my patients know that I am still here to support them, them and that the **referral is simply an extension of their care**, not a dismissal of their needs.

The referral process should be **seamless**, with clear communication between me and the specialist involved. I make it a point to provide a comprehensive report to the referring doctor, detailing the patient's medical history, treatments, and progress so far. This ensures that the patient does not have to repeat themselves or undergo unnecessary tests.

Additionally, I encourage patients to seek a second opinion if they feel it is necessary. The goal is never to limit their options but to ensure they are receiving the care that is best suited to their specific condition. If a patient feels more comfortable with a second opinion, I fully support that decision, as it leads to a greater sense of empowerment and confidence in their treatment journey.

Building a Supportive Network

The role of referrals and second opinions is not just about individual patient care—it's about creating a

network of professionals working together to provide the most holistic care possible. When I refer a patient to another healthcare provider, I know that this collaborative approach increases the chances of **positive outcomes**.

At the same time, patients should feel that they have a **partnership** in their healthcare. My role as a pain specialist is not to impose a single course of treatment but to empower the patient by offering them choices. Referrals and second opinions are part of this process. I want them to know that they make the most important health decisions, and I am here to help through every step.

Conclusion

The journey to pain relief is rarely a straightforward path. It's a journey that may involve multiple perspectives, varied expertise, and different approaches. By embracing referrals and second opinions as part of the collaborative process, we ensure that the patient receives the most **comprehensive**, **personalized**, and **effective** care possible. In order to give every patient the best chance of healing, I sometimes need to recognize when another expert is necessary. Ultimately, the most important thing is that the patient feels supported, heard, and confident in their treatment plan—no matter how many specialists it takes to achieve that. After all, **the best outcome for our patients is always worth the effort it takes to seek the best care possible**.

Chapter - 6

Bridging Gaps In Patient Communication

6.1 Overcoming Language and Cultural Barriers

As a pain specialist, I have come to understand that treating pain goes beyond just prescribing medications or performing procedures. A key aspect of healing is **communication**—and this becomes especially important when patients come from diverse linguistic and cultural backgrounds. When patients cannot express their pain, concerns, or needs clearly, it not only complicates their treatment but can also hinder their healing process. Overcoming **language** and **cultural barriers** is essential in providing holistic care and fostering a trusting doctor-patient relationship.

The Role of Language in Pain Management

Language is more than just words. It's how we **connect**, how we convey our **experiences**, and how we share what we're going through. Pain is a deeply personal experience, and without the right words to describe it, patients often feel misunderstood. Miscommunication can frustrate both the patient and the doctor, especially if the patient struggles to describe their pain.

I've seen firsthand in my practice how language can influence how people perceive and treat pain. When patients speak a language different from mine, there can be misunderstandings, even when using translation services. For example, some languages might lack specific words for certain sensations of pain, making it difficult for the patient to explain their symptoms accurately. In these instances, I rely heavily on **non-verbal cues**, like the patient's body language and facial expressions, to understand the intensity and nature of their pain.

But language barriers aren't just about vocabulary—they are also about **context**. Certain cultures may interpret the concept of pain differently. For instance, some communities view pain as something to endure silently, while others may be more open in expressing their suffering. A patient's attitude toward pain is shaped by **cultural** and **social norms**, and understanding these nuances is crucial for providing care that respects their values and beliefs.

Strategies for Overcoming Language Barriers

When language barriers exist, my primary goal is to ensure that the patient **feels heard** and understood. I've found several strategies that help bridge the communication gap:

1. **Use of Professional Interpreters**: One of the most effective tools is employing trained interpreters who can translate medical terms accurately. This helps ensure that the patient's concerns are conveyed properly and that the doctor's instructions are clearly

understood. I always prefer using **medical interpreters** over family members to avoid any potential inaccuracies in translation.

2. **Simplifying Medical Language**: Medical jargon can be overwhelming, especially when patients are dealing with pain and emotional stress. I make it a point to **simplify language** and avoid complex medical terms unless absolutely necessary. I explain things in layman's terms to ensure that the patient fully understands their diagnosis, treatment options, and the steps they need to take for recovery.

3. **Visual Aids**: Sometimes, the most effective way to communicate is not through words at all. I use **visual aids**, diagrams, and illustrations to explain the anatomy of pain or the mechanics of a treatment plan. These visual cues can be especially helpful for patients who may struggle to understand medical terms or for those with limited language proficiency.

4. **Patient Education Materials**: Providing written materials in the patient's preferred language ensures that they have a clear reference to go back to. These materials can include brochures, instructions for medication, and educational content about pain management.

5. **Technology**: In today's digital world, there are various apps and platforms that facilitate communication between patients and doctors, even if they don't share a common language. Some apps provide instant translation, while others allow for video consultations with interpreters. I embrace

these technologies when necessary, as they can be invaluable tools for bridging the language gap.

Cultural Sensitivity in Pain Management

Despite language barriers, cultural differences significantly influence the experience, expression, and management of pain. **Cultural competence** is an essential skill for me as a healthcare provider, especially in a diverse country where patients come from a wide variety of ethnic, religious, and socio-economic backgrounds. Being sensitive to cultural differences can help me build trust, demonstrate respect, and provide care that is not only effective but also aligned with the patient's values.

For example, some cultures may prioritize alternative therapies such as **herbal remedies**, **acupuncture**, or **spiritual healing** over conventional medical treatments. As a pain specialist, it's essential for me to **respect these preferences** and, when appropriate, work collaboratively with patients to integrate these practices with scientifically backed pain management techniques.

Similarly, different cultures have varying expectations about the **doctor-patient relationship**. In some cultures, patients may feel more comfortable with a paternalistic model of care, where the doctor makes most of the decisions. In contrast, others may prefer a more collaborative approach, approach where the patient is actively involved in decision-making. Understanding these cultural preferences helps me tailor my approach to meet the patient's needs while fostering a sense of autonomy and respect.

Addressing the Psychological and Emotional Aspects of Pain

Language and cultural barriers affect how we talk about, perceive, and respond to pain Cultural expectations often magnify the psychological and emotional aspects of pain. For instance, in some cultures, admitting to feeling vulnerable or needing emotional support might be seen as a weakness, leading patients to bottle up their emotions. This can worsen the impact of chronic pain.

On the other hand, some cultures may place a high value on **family** and **community support**. For these patients, involving family members in the care process is crucial for their healing journey. I take care to include the patient's family, if they desire, in discussions about treatment plans, pain management strategies, and recovery goals.

I also encourage patients to express not only their physical symptoms but also any emotional challenges they may be experiencing as a result of their pain. Whether it's feelings of **frustration**, **hopelessness**, or **anxiety**, acknowledging these emotions can play a pivotal role in pain management. Understanding the **emotional** aspects of pain helps me provide a more comprehensive treatment plan that includes both **physical** and **psychological support**.

Culturally Tailored Pain Management Plans

Ultimately, overcoming language and cultural barriers isn't just about translating words; it's about fostering **mutual understanding** and creating a treatment plan that takes into account both the **biological** and **cultural** dimensions of pain. Every patient is unique, and their cultural background plays a significant role in how they experience and cope with pain.

By recognizing and respecting these differences, I can help create **personalized** and **culturally sensitive pain management plans** that are more likely to resonate with the patient and lead to better outcomes. This holistic approach to pain management not only enhances the patient's **physical well-being** but also improves their overall sense of **empowerment**, **dignity**, and **self-worth**.

Conclusion

Pain management is as much about communication as it is about treatment. Overcoming language and cultural barriers requires patience, empathy, and a commitment to providing care that acknowledges and respects the patient's background. Whether it's using interpreters, simplifying medical language, or incorporating culturally relevant practices, my goal is always the same: to ensure that the patient feels **heard**, **understood**, and **supported** on their journey to recovery.

Cultural competence is a fundamental aspect of providing exceptional care in a world that is becoming increasingly diverse. By embracing the diversity of the patients I serve, I can help them achieve not just relief from pain, pain but also a sense of **dignity**, **respect**, and **hope**.

6.2 Using Data and Technology to Enhance Doctor-Patient Interaction

In today's fast-paced medical world, the integration of **data** and **technology** has transformed how we approach patient care, especially in pain management. As a pain specialist, I've witnessed the remarkable benefits that data-driven tools and technology offer in improving the quality of doctor-patient interactions. These advancements enable me to **better understand patient needs**, provide more **personalized care**, and ensure **ongoing communication**—all of which ultimately lead to more effective treatment outcomes.

The Role of Data in Pain Management

Data is the cornerstone of modern medicine. With the rise of **electronic health records (EHRs)**, **patient monitoring devices**, and **pain tracking apps**, we have access to a wealth of information that can help guide our decisions. In my practice, I rely heavily on data to **track pain levels**, monitor patient progress, and adjust treatment plans accordingly.

Pain is subjective—what one patient experiences as excruciating, another might describe as tolerable. However, with the help of **digital pain diaries** and **pain tracking apps**, we can measure pain in a more **quantifiable** manner. These tools allow patients to log their pain levels in real time, offering a more accurate picture of their pain patterns and triggers. Patients can also record other factors such as sleep quality, mood, and medication use, giving us a holistic view of how pain impacts their daily lives.

By regularly reviewing this data, I can identify trends or patterns that may have gone unnoticed during a traditional office visit. This helps me adjust treatment plans more effectively and intervene earlier if necessary. For instance, if a patient reports that their pain is worsening at certain times of the day or after specific activities, we can tailor their therapy to target those specific triggers.

Technology for Remote Monitoring and Communication

One of the most profound changes in healthcare over the past decade has been the shift to telemedicine. Through virtual consultations, patients no longer have to wait for a physical appointment to discuss their progress or concerns. They can now speak to me from the comfort of their homes, no matter where they are located.

Telemedicine has facilitated access to specialized care for patients, particularly those residing in rural or remote areas. For many, having a consultation without the need to travel can significantly improve their quality of life. In pain management, this is particularly important. Many patients with chronic pain struggle with mobility and find it difficult to leave the house for appointments. Virtual visits remove this barrier and allow for continuous, uninterrupted care.

Additionally, through **remote monitoring devices**, we can track various metrics such as heart rate, blood pressure, and even muscle tension. These devices can alert me in real time if a patient is experiencing unusual symptoms or if their pain levels are escalating, enabling me to intervene immediately and adjust their care plan without requiring an in-person visit.

Artificial Intelligence and Machine Learning in Pain Assessment

The introduction of **artificial intelligence (AI)** and **machine learning** in healthcare has made a significant impact on pain management. These technologies can analyze vast amounts of data quickly and accurately, identifying patterns that may be invisible to the human eye. In my practice, I use AI-powered tools to help with **diagnosis** and **treatment decisions**.

For example, **AI algorithms** can analyze pain reports, medical history, and other diagnostic data to suggest personalized treatment options based on a patient's unique profile. This allows me to offer more **precise** and **targeted** therapies, increasing the likelihood of effective pain relief.

Machine learning can also help in identifying **predictive markers** for pain progression. By looking at historical data, these tools can forecast which patients are at higher risk for developing chronic pain or experiencing flare-ups. This helps me proactively manage their treatment and potentially prevent the worsening of their condition.

Patient Portals : Enhancing Communication and Empowerment

In many healthcare settings today, **patient portals** have become an essential part of patient interaction. These online platforms allow patients to **view their medical records**, **request prescriptions**, and **schedule**

appointments with ease. For me, patient portals are a valuable tool that enhances communication and keeps patients involved in their own care.

Patients can access detailed information about their treatment plan, track their pain levels, and even send secure messages to me with questions or updates about their condition. This eliminates the need for phone calls and long waiting times to get answers, which can be especially frustrating for patients in chronic pain. Having the ability to communicate directly with their doctor in real time can significantly improve their overall experience and reduce feelings of **helplessness**.

Moreover, patient portals allow for **better patient education**. I can upload resources about pain management, exercises, nutrition, and self-care strategies that patients can refer to at their convenience. This empowers patients to take an active role in their healing journey, providing them with the tools and knowledge they need to manage their pain more effectively.

The Promise of Personalized Pain Management

What excites me the most about the future of pain management is the potential to move toward **personalized care**. With the help of data and technology, we are now able to create more individualized treatment plans that take into account not just the patient's medical history but also their lifestyle, preferences, and even genetics.

For example, with genetic testing, we can better understand how a patient's body metabolizes certain medications, allowing us to choose the **most effective pain relief options** with fewer side effects. This minimizes the trial-and-error process and helps patients find relief faster.

In addition, **wearable devices** and **smart sensors** can continuously track real-time data, allowing us to monitor a patient's pain levels and adjust treatment in a more **dynamic** way. By combining all of this information—data from tracking apps, remote monitoring, AI-driven insights, and genetic testing—we can offer truly **customized pain relief** that is far more effective than the one-size-fits-all approaches of the past.

Improving the Doctor-Patient Relationship

While technology offers immense potential for improving patient care, it's important to remember that at the heart of any treatment is the **doctor-patient relationship**. Data and technology should **enhance**, not replace, human connection. I still take the time to listen to my patients, understand their concerns, and make them feel seen and heard. Technology should be seen as a tool that helps me provide **better care**, but the foundation of that care is still rooted in empathy and communication.

By using data and technology, I am able to be more **efficient**, **informed**, and **responsive** to my patients' needs. However, it is the trust and rapport built through personal interaction that allow me to truly make a difference in their lives.

Conclusion

The integration of **data** and **technology** into pain management has revolutionized the way we approach patient care. By using tools like pain tracking apps, remote monitoring devices, AI, and patient portals, I am able to offer **personalized**, **precise**, and **continuous** care to my patients, enhancing the doctor-patient relationship and improving treatment outcomes. However, it is essential that we use these tools thoughtfully and always remember that the ultimate goal is to provide care that is **compassionate**, **empowering**, and centered on the patient's **individual needs**.

In this digital age, the future of pain management is both **exciting** and **transformative**. By embracing technology, we can provide a superior level of care and guarantee that no patient experiences their pain journey alone

6.3 Simplifying complex diagnoses for patients

As a pain specialist, one of the most critical aspects of my work is ensuring that my patients understand their diagnosis clearly and without confusion. Complex underlying causes often accompany chronic pain, and a difficult diagnosis can overwhelm patients. The medical terminology, the range of tests, and the uncertainty surrounding treatment options can leave patients feeling lost and unsure of what steps to take next. That's where **clear communication** becomes vital.

Over the years, I've learned that **simplifying complex diagnoses** is not just about making the medical language easier to understand—it's about empowering the patient with knowledge so they can make informed decisions about their care. It's about breaking down the complicated aspects of their condition and putting it into terms they can relate to, all while maintaining the integrity of the medical facts.

The Power of Analogies and Visual Aids

One of the most effective tools I use in my practice is **analogies**. Making a comparison between a complex medical concept and something familiar to the patient can significantly impact their understanding.

For example, when explaining **nerve damage** in conditions like **sciatica**, I might compare the nerve to an electrical wire. Fraying or damage to the wire causes the signal to misfire, leading to pain or numbness. This analogy helps the patient visualize what's happening in their body without feeling overwhelmed by technical jargon.

In addition to analogies, **visual aids** such as diagrams, charts, or even 3D models have proven to be incredibly helpful. They allow me to visually show patients where the problem is located in their body and how it's affecting their function. For instance, I often use models of the spine to explain how **herniated discs** might compress nerves and lead to pain. **Interactive tools**, like digital imaging, allow the patient to explore the parts of their body that are involved in their pain, which can improve their understanding and engagement in the treatment process.

Breaking Down Medical Jargon

Another common challenge is the use of **medical jargon**. Many patients, understandably, are not familiar with terms like **radiculopathy**, **spondylosis**, or **neuropathy**, and this can create a barrier to understanding. To combat this, I make a conscious effort to break down each term into simpler, everyday language. Instead of saying "Your MRI shows evidence of a herniated disc causing radiculopathy," I would say, "The MRI shows that a disc in your spine is pushing on a nerve, which is causing pain to travel down your leg."

By **rephrasing** medical terms and using language that feels more approachable, patients are able to grasp the meaning of their diagnosis with less anxiety. Instead of hearing a foreign language, they now receive explanations that align with their own understanding.

Engaging Patients in Their Diagnosis

I also make sure to involve patients in their own diagnosis process. This involves encouraging patients to ask questions, voice their concerns, and participate in the decision-making process.

Patients often feel like the doctor is telling them what to do without being involved. But in my experience, patients are more likely to adhere to a treatment plan when they understand it and feel involved in the decision-making.

I always ensure that I explain **why** certain tests are necessary, what they are looking for, and how the results will influence treatment decisions. For example, if a patient is undergoing nerve conduction studies to check for nerve damage, I explain the purpose of the test, what the sensations they experience during it might mean, and how the results will help guide treatment options. This process not only clarifies the diagnosis but also builds trust between the patient and me as their physician.

The Importance of Emotional Support

Diagnosing chronic pain is often a difficult process, and many patients may struggle with feelings of **frustration** and **helplessness** when faced with a diagnosis that requires long-term management. Therefore, **emotional support** plays a vital role in simplifying complex diagnoses. When I share the results of a test or imaging study with a patient, I make sure to explain the diagnosis clearly, but I also offer support and encouragement. For instance, I reassure them that while the path to healing may be long, there are numerous treatment options and a team of professionals ready to help.

When a patient is feeling overwhelmed, I offer to break down the information step-by-step, ensuring they don't feel rushed. I also encourage them to bring a **family member or friend** to appointments so they can have someone there for emotional and logistical support. This sense of shared understanding can be comforting as patients begin to navigate their diagnosis.

Creating a Roadmap for the Patient

A diagnosis can often feel like a starting point with no clear path forward. This is especially true in the realm of chronic pain, where a variety of treatment options and adjustments may be required. In these cases, I take time to create a **personalized roadmap** for the patient. This roadmap not only explains their diagnosis but also breaks down the **steps** they can take to manage and alleviate their pain.

For example, if the patient has been diagnosed with **osteoarthritis**, I would walk them through the treatment options, from **physical therapy** and **lifestyle changes** to **medication management** and, if necessary, **injections** or **surgical procedures**. I clearly outline what they can expect from each step, the timeframe for potential improvement, and any lifestyle adjustments they may need to make along the way.

This roadmap gives patients something tangible to hold onto. They see that there is a plan and that their journey has steps, not an unknown path. It empowers them and gives them back some sense of control in what may feel like an uncontrollable situation.

Building Trust through Transparent Communication

One of the most important aspects of simplifying complex diagnoses is **building trust** through transparent communication. When patients feel that they are receiving clear, honest, and understandable information, they are more likely to trust the doctor's expertise and feel more confident in the treatment decisions being made. This trust is foundational to successful treatment outcomes, particularly in the case of chronic pain, where long-term management is required.

Every patient is unique, and I make sure to tailor my explanations to fit each individual's needs, ensuring they understand their diagnosis and the path forward. More than simplifying information, it empowers patients to actively participate in their care.

Conclusion

Simplifying complex diagnoses is about more than just breaking down medical jargon—it's about ensuring that patients understand their condition, feel empowered to make informed decisions, and receive the support they need to move forward. By using clear language, visual aids, analogies, and creating personalized roadmaps, we can enhance the doctor-patient relationship and make the journey through chronic pain more manageable. With patience, empathy, and clear communication, we can make even the most complicated diagnoses feel more approachable, providing our patients with the clarity they deserve.

6.4 The Art of Listening: Why It's Critical

As a doctor, I have always believed that **listening** is one of the most essential skills in my practice. Pain, especially chronic pain, is deeply personal. Every patient brings their own experience, their own story, and their own struggles with them to the clinic. **Listening** is not

just about hearing what they say—it's about truly understanding the emotions, frustrations, and fears behind their words.

The act of listening often gets lost in the chaos of daily appointments and the pressure to solve complex problems. But in my experience, **attentive listening** is at the core of effective pain management. Building trust and gaining deeper insights into a patient's condition hinges on attentive listening.

The Power of Active Listening

Active listening goes beyond simply hearing the words spoken by a patient. It involves giving the patient your **undivided attention**, making eye contact, and focusing on what they are saying without interrupting. Respond in a way that shows you understand their words, emotions, and contextI pay attention to the tone of their voice, the pace of their speech, and even their body language when I actively listen.I can often sense when a patient is holding back or when they're unsure about something. These subtle cues can reveal more than the words themselves and provide important insights into the emotional and psychological aspects of their pain. This deeper understanding can lead to better diagnoses and more personalized treatment plans.

For example, when a patient describes their pain as "stabbing" or "shooting," these words might give me clues about the **nerve involvement**. But when they say, "It feels like my whole body is exhausted from fighting it," that might indicate a **deeper emotional burden**, like stress or anxiety, contributing to the pain.

Building Trust Through Empathy

When patients feel truly heard, they begin to trust their healthcare provider more deeply. **Empathy** plays a vital role here. Instead of nodding and agreeing, put yourself in the patient's shoes and acknowledge their pain. I've found that simply saying, "I understand how this must be so difficult for you" or "I can see how frustrating this must be" can be incredibly reassuring.

Empathy helps build a **stronger doctor-patient relationship**, one based on mutual respect and understanding. Patients feel more comfortable sharing the details of their pain and health when they receive attention and validation for their concerns.

This creates a space where open communication can thrive, and we can work together to find solutions.

For example, if a patient is dealing with **chronic back pain** and feels that no one has truly listened to their experience, I make sure to validate their emotions. Sometimes the pain extends beyond physical boundaries, affecting their sense of identity, their ability to work, or their role in the family.

Acknowledging these aspects helps the patient feel seen and understood.

The Patient's Narrative: Key to Diagnosis

Pain, particularly chronic pain, often has a **narrative**—a story that evolves over time. Everyone's pain story, how it's affected their life, and how they've managed it is different. By listening closely to this narrative, I can gain critical insights into the **root causes** of their condition and how it has impacted them on a deeper level.

For example, a patient might describe how their pain started after a **sports injury**, but over time, it worsened and began affecting their mood, relationships, and daily activities. As they share their story, I listen not only to the physical aspects but also to the emotional and psychological factors at play. Pain often has multiple layers—physical, emotional, and mental. The more I listen to the full narrative, the more I understand the complete picture of what my patient is going through. By engaging in this **storytelling process**, I can better tailor the treatment to fit the patient's **needs**. It's not just about alleviating physical pain—it's about improving quality of life, managing stress, and addressing the emotional aspects of chronic pain. Connecting the physical and emotional components of pain through listening enables more comprehensive care.

Listening to Understand, Not to Respond

As doctors, we often have a tendency to swiftly evaluate the issue, provide a diagnosis, and recommend a treatment plan. But in doing so, we may miss out on important details that could change the course of treatment.

In my practice, I remind myself to **listen to understand**, not just to respond. Sometimes, the patient just needs to express their frustrations, fears, or anxieties without interruption. Often, after they've spoken, they feel lighter, more understood, and more ready to hear treatment options. In those moments, I realize that the simple act of listening has already begun the healing process.

There are times when a patient doesn't need immediate answers but simply a space to **express themselves**. By giving them that space, I show them that their experience matters, that I am here to listen, and that we are inon this journey together.

Breaking Down Barriers in Communication

The fear of not understanding or believing is one of the biggest barriers in doctor-patient communication. This fear is particularly prevalent among those suffering from chronic pain. Especially when their pain is difficult to diagnose or treat, many patients report feeling dismissed or ignored by previous healthcare providers. Listening allows me to **break down these barriers**. When I ask open-ended questions and give patients the time and space to speak freely, they begin to open up about their experiences. This fosters a secure atmosphere where patients feel their pain is receiving serious attention. It also guarantees that I avoid hasty judgments and instead gather all the necessary information for a precise diagnosis. When a patient feels that their concerns have been heard, they are more likely to trust the treatment recommendations that follow. Patients are more inclined to adhere to their care plan and experience a renewed sense of hope for effective pain management.

Improving Treatment Outcomes

The impact of truly listening to patients extends far beyond just building rapport—it can **significantly improve treatment outcomes**. When I actively listen, I am better equipped to understand the full spectrum of their pain, not just its physical symptoms but also the emotional and social factors contributing to their condition. This comprehensive understanding allows me to design more **personalized treatment plans**, addressing not just the symptoms but the root causes of pain.

For example, if a patient is dealing with **chronic knee pain**, pain but also mentions that their pain worsens when they are stressed or anxious, I may incorporate **stress management techniques** or suggest **mental health support** alongside physical treatments. Understanding the full scope of a patient's pain—physical and emotional—can lead to better outcomes and a more effective treatment plan.

Conclusion: Listening as a Lifelong Practice

It takes a lifetime to master the art of listening. As doctors, we must continually remind ourselves that our patients are not just cases to solve but people with their own struggles and stories. By truly listening, we can uncover the nuances of their pain, address the emotional factors at play, and create more meaningful, effective treatment plans.

Ultimately, listening is a tool that builds trust, improves communication, and leads to better outcomes. It is a simple yet profound way to show patients that they are not alone in their pain—that we, as healthcare providers, are here to walk alongside them in their journey toward healing.

6.5 Handling Unrealistic Expectations Compassionately

As a doctor, one of the most delicate challenges I face is managing **unrealistic expectations** about pain relief and treatment outcomes. It's not uncommon for patients to come to me with **high hopes** for a quick fix—especially when they've suffered for years and are desperate for a solution. They may have heard success stories from others or even seen advertisements promising instant results, leading them to believe that relief is just a prescription away.

But the reality is: pain is complex. It doesn't always follow a predictable path, and sometimes, even the most advanced treatments take time to show results. The key to handling these expectations compassionately lies in the way we **communicate** with our patients. **Compassionate care** means recognizing their fears, frustrations, and hopes, hopes while gently guiding them toward a realistic understanding of their condition and treatment options.

Understanding the Root of Unrealistic Expectations

Unrealistic expectations often stem from **misinformation**, **misunderstandings**, or **previous failed experiences**. Patients may have been told by others that a specific treatment or therapy will "cure" them in a matter of days. This can create anthe illusion that all they need is the right intervention, and everything will improve immediately. In many cases, it's not that the patient is unwilling to accept the reality of their pain, but rather that they are hoping for a **quick solution** to relieve their suffering.

When a patient expresses frustration or anxiety about their treatment not working as quickly as they expected, I try to acknowledge those emotions first. It's important to empathize with their **disappointment** and **desperation**, and then gently help them understand the nature of their pain. This compassionate approach cultivates trust and creates a constructive dialogue about achievable goals.

Setting Realistic Goals Together

One of the most powerful ways to manage unrealistic expectations is to work **collaboratively** with patients to set **realistic goals**. Rather than offering vague promises, I believe in breaking down the treatment process into smaller, more manageable steps. This not only helps the patient see progress but also provides them with a sense of agency and control over their healing journey.

For example, if a patient comes in with the expectation that a single session of physical therapy will completely eliminate their pain, I would explain that while therapy can be incredibly effective, it is most often a **long-term process** that requires consistent effort. I would work with the patient to outline a **timeline** for recovery and create a plan that includes both **short-term goals** (such as reducing pain intensity) and **long-term goals** (such as improving mobility and function). By breaking things down, we can align their expectations with what's actually possible within a given timeframe.

Education and Communication

Education is an essential part of managing unrealistic expectations. It's important to **inform patients** about the chronic nature of some pain conditions and how treatment works over time. Many chronic pain conditions, such as osteoarthritis or fibromyalgia, require ongoing management rather than one-time cures. Educating patients about the science behind their condition and the steps involved in their treatment allows them to better understand that **healing** often involves a **multifaceted approach** that includes medication, physical therapy, lifestyle changes, and sometimes, sometimes emotional support.

For instance, I may explain that **inflammation** and **nerve damage** can take months to heal and that consistent therapy can gradually improve their symptoms. I also emphasize the importance of **patience** and **self-care** practices in managing their condition. This helps patients feel more **empowered** and less frustrated by the process. It's also crucial to explain that setbacks are a natural part of the journey, and progress might be slow but steady.

Addressing Emotional Needs

Sometimes, unrealistic expectations stem from deeper **emotional needs**—such as fear, anxiety, or feelings of helplessness. Chronic pain not only burdens the body physically, but also emotionally. Patients may fear that their pain will never end, end or that it will impact their ability to live their lives fully. These emotional aspects can cloud their judgment and make them cling to the idea of a quick fix.

In such cases, I make sure to offer a **supportive and reassuring** presence. I tell my patients that it's okay to feel frustrated, but that **healing** is a process, and while it may be difficult, they are not alone. Compassionate listening plays a huge role here—when a patient feels heard and understood, they are more likely to open up about their emotional concerns.

By acknowledging and addressing these emotions, I can build a deeper rapport with my patients and help them set more realistic, achievable goals. It's also important to remind them that **mental health** plays a significant role in pain management, and it's okay to seek **emotional support** through counseling, stress management, or support groups.

Providing Options and Alternatives

Another effective strategy for managing unrealistic expectations is offering **alternative treatment options**. Patients often come to me expecting a single solution, such as surgery or a prescription medication, to fix their pain. While these options can be helpful, they may not always be the best fit, especially for chronic conditions. By discussing a **variety of approaches**, including physical therapy, lifestyle modifications, supplements, or mental health support, I can offer patients a more comprehensive treatment plan that addresses multiple aspects of their pain.

For example, if a patient insists that they want an immediate solution like a strong painkiller or surgery, I'll gently explain that while those treatments can be effective, they often don't address the underlying causes of pain in the long run. Instead, I might suggest **a combination of therapies** that promote healing in the body, like physical therapy, exercise, and mindfulness. This empowers the patient to take a more holistic approach to managing their pain, pain rather than relying on quick fixes that might not offer lasting relief.

Reinforcing Progress and Celebrating Small Wins

Finally, it's important to **reinforce any progress**—even small milestones—as patients move through their treatment journey. Often, patients who expect rapid results feel discouraged if their pain doesn't disappear immediately. I make sure to celebrate small victories, such as a decrease in pain intensity, an improvement in mobility, or even a better mood. These small wins can be incredibly motivating and help patients see that they are making progress, even if it feels slow.

For instance, if a patient who has been struggling with knee pain for years reports that they can walk for 20 minutes without pain, I make sure to acknowledge that achievement. It's a reminder that while **full relief** may take time, they are on the right path.

Conclusion: Compassionate Realism

Handling unrealistic expectations is a delicate balance between **compassion** and **realism**. As a doctor, my role is to guide patients through the complex landscape of pain management with both empathy and practical knowledge. By listening, educating, and setting achievable goals, we can help patients manage their expectations and find realistic paths to relief. It's a journey, not a race, and with compassionate care, patience, and persistence, we can walk with our patients every step of the way

Chapter - 7

Beyond Pills And Procedures

7.1 Why a Quick Fix Rarely Works

As a doctor, one of the most common misconceptions I encounter is the belief that a **quick fix** is the ultimate solution to chronic pain. Many patients seek immediate relief from me, often hoping for a magic pill, an instant procedure, or a simple answer that will permanently eliminate their pain. I understand the **desperation** that comes from living with constant discomfort, and while I deeply empathize with that, it's essential to recognize that **pain management**—especially for chronic conditions—is not about finding an instant fix.

I always remind my patients that pain, particularly chronic pain, is often **multifactorial**, meaning it arises from multiple sources, including **physical, emotional**, and **psychological** factors. Just as pain doesn't develop overnight, it cannot be solved with a **quick fix**. In fact, seeking rapid relief may provide only **temporary results**, leaving the underlying causes of pain untreated.

The Illusion of Instant Relief

The allure of a quick fix is strong. There are plenty of treatments out there—whether it's an over-the-counter painkiller, an injection, or a one-time procedure—that promise immediate relief. And while these can sometimes offer temporary respite, they rarely address the root causes of pain. It's important to understand that **pain is a symptom**, not a disease in itself. It is a signal that something deeper needs attention. Focusing solely on eliminating the sensation of pain without understanding its origin is like putting a **band-aid** on a wound that requires stitches.

Take painkillers, for instance. They might **mask** the discomfort for a while, but they don't fix the underlying **inflammation**, **nerve damage**, or **muscle imbalances** that could be the true culprits. Similarly, procedures like **joint injections** or **spinal surgeries** can provide temporary relief but are not always a permanent solution. These interventions don't address the overall **health** and **well-being** of the body.

Chronic Pain Needs a Holistic Approach

In my practice, I have seen countless patients who arrive with the expectation that **one treatment** will completely resolve their pain. But the reality is, managing chronic pain requires a **holistic approach**—a plan that involves multiple strategies to address the **physical**, **mental**, and **emotional** aspects of pain.

For example, consider **arthritis**. The physical wear and tear on the joints can cause pain, but there may also be an emotional component tied to the experience of living with a chronic condition. A **multi-faceted treatment plan** that includes not just medication or surgery, surgery but also **physical therapy**, **nutritional support**, and **stress management** can lead to far better, more sustainable outcomes.

In many cases, physical therapy and exercise play a critical role. Exercise helps strengthen the muscles around the affected joints, relieving stress on the bones and improving mobility. But it's not just about physical treatments—**nutrition** plays a huge role in inflammation, and **mental health** plays a significant part in how we perceive and cope with pain.

The Role of Patience and Consistency

One of the most important lessons I've learned in my years of practice is that **patience** and **consistency** are crucial for managing chronic pain. It's not easy, and it's certainly not a quick fix. But with the right approach, we can significantly improve the quality of life and reduce pain levels over time.

When patients start a new treatment plan, they often expect results within the first few days or weeks. However, healing takes time. This is particularly true for conditions like **chronic back pain**, **fibromyalgia**, or **migraines**, which may require several months of **regular treatment** and **lifestyle changes** before significant relief is felt. That's why I emphasize the importance of **commitment** to the process. Whether it's a specific exercise regimen, dietary changes, or mental health strategies, results often come gradually. The key is **consistency**—continuing to follow the plan even when immediate relief is not apparent.

I always tell my patients that it's like tending to a garden. You plant the seeds of beneficial habits—be it through therapy, exercise, or nutrition—and you nurture them over time.

You don't expect the flowers to bloom overnight. But with patience, care, and persistence, the results will come.

The Problem with the "Quick-Fix" Mentality

The problem with the **quick-fix mentality** is that it often leads to **disappointment** and **frustration** when the desired results don't occur immediately. Patients might experience a sense of defeat, believing that the treatment is ineffective or they will forever endure pain. They might then resort to **more invasive procedures** or **medications**, hoping that something stronger will work. This creates a cycle of frustration, as each quick fix temporarily alleviates symptoms but doesn't heal the body or mind in the long run.

Moreover, many quick fixes—especially those involving medications or invasive procedures—can come with significant **side effects** and **risks**. Medications can lead to **dependency**, surgeries carry inherent risks, and procedures like injections can have limited effectiveness over time. Relying too heavily on these solutions can trap patients in a cycle of seeking immediate relief without addressing the larger picture.

Empowering Patients for Long-Term Relief

Thus, the goal is to relieve pain immediately and empower patients to manage it long-term. I always encourage my patients to become **active participants** in their healing journey. This entails committing to a treatment plan that incorporates a variety of therapies, lifestyle modifications, and emotional support. It also means being **realistic** about expectations, expectations and understanding that true healing takes time and dedication.

For example, in cases of **chronic knee pain**, rather than immediately turning to surgery, we focus on strengthening the surrounding muscles, improving flexibility, and reducing inflammation through diet and exercise. This multi-pronged approach not only relieves pain but also helps improve function, providing lasting benefits rather than temporary relief.

Conclusion: Patiencepatience, Persistencepersistance, and Personalizationpersonnalisation

Ultimately, **pain management** is not about finding a **quick fix**, fix but about finding the right solutions that will work **for you** over time. Every patient is different, and it's essential to develop a **personalized treatment plan** that addresses your specific needs, lifestyle, and goals. While a quick fix may sound appealing, it's often only a temporary solution, whereas a comprehensive, holistic approach can lead to long-term relief and a higher quality of life.

As a doctor, I'm here to guide you on this journey, helping you to understand the full scope of your condition and working with you to find the best, most sustainable solutions. Together, we can build a path forward that goes beyond pills and procedures and empowers you to take charge of your pain, your health, and your life.

7.2 Identifying Your Pain Triggers

One of the most powerful tools in managing chronic pain is **awareness**—specifically, the ability to identify what triggers or exacerbates your pain. As a doctor, I often see patients who struggle with the unpredictabilityunpredictable nature of their pain. Pain can fluctuate, sometimes without a clear cause, leaving patients feeling frustrated and helpless.

But the reality is, **pain triggers** are often present, and learning to identify them is key to not only managing pain but also **preventing flare-ups**.

Pain is a complex experience, and no two people's pain triggers are exactly the same. This is why understanding your own unique pain triggers is so important. It's about creating a **personalized roadmap** to help you navigate your condition and **minimize discomfort** in your day-to-day life.

What Are Pain Triggers?

Pain triggers are specific factors or situations that **increase** or **worsen** your pain. These triggers could be **physical**, **emotional**, or **environmental** in nature, and they vary greatly from person to person. For example, a person with **migraines** may experience an episode after exposure to bright lights or strong smells, while someone with **chronic back pain** might find that long periods of sitting or standing worsen their symptoms.

Triggers can also be **psychological**—stress, anxiety, or negative emotions can amplify pain perception.

Deep interconnection exists between the mind and body, with one often influencing the other. This is why **understanding your pain triggers** involves paying attention to both physical sensations and your emotional state.

Common Pain Triggers

Over the years, I've found that most patients can identify several common triggers for their pain, even if they don't immediately recognize them. Some of these include:

- **Physical Activity**: Sometimes, overexertion or certain movements can cause pain to flare. This is common for those dealing with joint pain, **muscle strains**, or even conditions like **fibromyalgia**. On the other hand, a **lack of movement** can also exacerbate pain, particularly in conditions like **arthritis**.

- **Stress**: Emotional stress can have a profound impact on pain levels. The body's **stress response** can cause muscles to tense up, which in turn increases pain, especially in areas like the **neck**, **back**, and **shoulders**. Chronic stress can also trigger **inflammation**, worsening conditions like **rheumatoid arthritis**.

- **Dietary Choices**: Certain foods may inflame or trigger pain in some people. For example, foods that are high in **sugar**, **processed oils**, or **refined carbohydrates** can increase **inflammation**, making joint pain or conditions like **gout** worse. Conversely, **anti-inflammatory foods** like omega-3 fatty acids or antioxidants can help reduce pain levels.

- **Sleep Patterns**: Poor sleep is another common pain trigger. Lack of restorative sleep can make pain worse, leading to a vicious cycle where pain interrupts sleep, and poor sleep makes pain more intense. Conditions like **chronic fatigue syndrome** or **fibromyalgia** are often aggravated by inadequate rest.

- **Weather Changes**: Many patients with conditions like **osteoarthritis** or **muscle pain** report that their symptoms intensify when the weather changes. This is often due to the barometric pressure shifts, which can affect joint function and **nerve sensitivity**.

- **Medications**: While pain medications provide temporary relief, they can sometimes lead to **dependency** or have side effects that can trigger other pain symptoms. In particular, **opioid medications** can cause **constipation**, which in turn can cause abdominal pain or discomfort.

The Power of Tracking Your Pain

One of the best ways to identify pain triggers is by **tracking** your symptoms. As a doctor, I recommend that my patients keep a **pain diary**. This simple but effective tool involves logging your daily pain levels, activities, diet, sleep, and emotional state. By keeping track of these details, you can start to notice patterns that point to specific triggers.

For example, you might notice that after a particularly stressful week at work, your back pain worsens. Or perhaps, perhaps you find that you're more likely to have a headache on days when you don't get enough sleep or when you skip your regular exercise routine. These insights are invaluable because they can help you **make adjustments** to avoid or manage those triggers more effectively.

When keeping a pain diary, try to include:

- **Pain level** (on a scale from 1 to 10)
- **Activities you did** (both physical and emotional)
- **Diet** (any foods or drinks that might have triggered your pain)
- **Sleep quality**
- **Medications** taken and their effects
- **Any stressors** you encountered that day

Over time, you'll build a comprehensive picture of your pain and the factors that influence it. Once we identify these triggers, we can collaborate to devise strategies to prevent, control, or mitigate them.

Recognizing Emotional and Psychological Triggers

Pain is not just a physical phenomenon; it has a psychological component as well. For many individuals, stress, anxiety, and depression can act as powerful pain triggers. In fact, there's a feedback loop in which pain can worsen emotional distress, and emotional distress can make pain feel even more intense.

For example, when people are **anxious**, their bodies tend to tense up, which can exacerbate muscle pain or joint stiffness. Negative emotions can also lead to **poor posture** or **less movement**, further aggravating physical pain. Similarly, a **depressed mood** can make it harder to engage in self-care, such as exercising or eating healthily, which in turn can lead to a worsening of pain symptoms.

It's crucial to acknowledge the **emotional** and **psychological triggers** and address them as part of your pain management plan. If you find that emotional factors are playing a significant rolc in your pain, consider engaging in **therapy**, **mindfulness practices**, or stress management techniques like **meditation** and **yoga**.

Creating a Strategy to Minimize Pain Triggers

Once you've identified your pain triggers, the next step is to **create a strategy** for minimizing them. This is where we, as a healthcare team, come in. Based on your pain diary and discussions with your doctor, we can help you develop a tailored plan to manage your triggers.

Here are a few steps you can take:

1. **Modify Daily Activities**: If you notice that certain physical activities trigger your pain, it may be time to **adjust your routine**. Perhaps this means incorporating more breaks, adjusting your posture, or changing your exercise regimen.

2. **Practice Stress Reduction**: Stress is one of the most common pain triggers, so learning how to manage it is crucial. Techniques like **meditation**, **breathing exercises**, and **mindfulness** can help regulate stress levels, potentially reducing pain.

3. **Optimize Nutrition**: If dietary triggers are identified, consider adjusting your **meal plan**. Avoid inflammatory foods and increase your intake of **anti-inflammatory** foods like leafy greens, fish, nuts, and seeds. Consulting with a **nutritionist** can also help in creating a diet plan that aligns with your pain management goals.

4. **Prioritize Sleep**: Ensure you are getting enough **restful sleep** each night. Establish a sleep routine, keep your bedroom cool and dark, and avoid screens before bedtime. Sleep hygiene can significantly affect your pain levels.

5. **Stay Active**: While it may seem counterintuitive, **regular exercise** can actually help reduce pain. It’s essential to find an activity that is gentle yet effective, such as **swimming**, **yoga**, or **tai chi**.

Conclusion: Your Pain, Your Journey

Identifying pain triggers is a crucial step toward regaining control over your pain. By recognizing what causes or worsens your symptoms, you can take proactive steps to minimize these triggers, making it easier to live your life on your terms. Keep in mind, this is a personal journey, and it may take time to fully understand your triggers and how to manage them effectively. But with patience, persistence, and the right tools, you can find relief and improve your overall quality of life. Remember, **pain management** is not about eradicating every trigger, trigger but learning how to navigate them with confidence and control.

7.3 Creating a Pain Management Toolkit

As a doctor, one of my key roles is to empower you to take charge of your pain. A **pain management toolkit** is not just a collection of medications or therapies, but a **personalized approach** that combines various strategies to manage, reduce, and even prevent pain. It's a **holistic** system that puts you at the center of your care, allowing you to make informed decisions about how to live your life despite pain. This toolkit becomes your companion on your journey toward a pain-free existence, providing you with practical tools that align with your lifestyle, your condition, and your preferences.

Understanding the Pain Management Toolkit

Think of your **pain management toolkit** as a set of resources and strategies you can rely on whenever you experience pain. Just as a mechanic has various tools for different tasks, your toolkit will contain different options—some for **immediate relief**, others for **long-term management**. The key is not to rely on just one method, method but to have multiple options at your disposal. By choosing the right tool for the situation, you'll learn what works best for you over time. Creating your toolkit begins with understanding **your pain**, **your lifestyle**, and **your goals**. Once we understand these, we can begin building your personalized toolkit.

1. Understanding Your Pain

Before adding anything to your toolkit, it's important to have a deep understanding of your pain. **What triggers it? When does it flare up? What makes it better or worse?** We will tailor a toolkit to your unique needs based on these questions. For example, if you experience joint pain after long periods of sitting, incorporating regular movement or **stretching exercises** into your routine can be a helpful addition.

If stress exacerbates your pain, including **relaxation techniques** or **mindfulness practices** will become vital parts of your toolkit. The first step is always a **clear diagnosis** and an understanding of the triggers and patterns in your pain.

2. Pain Relief Techniques: Immediate Tools

Immediate relief options are critical, especially when pain strikes unexpectedly or intensely. These tools aim to offer immediate, temporary alleviation, assisting you in regaining comfort and mastery over your symptoms.

- **Pain Medication**: Prescription or over-the-counter medications can be an essential part of your toolkit.

NSAIDs (non-steroidal anti-inflammatory drugs) like ibuprofen or naproxen may be used for inflammatory pain. For some, **muscle relaxants** or **topical creams** (such as menthol or capsaicin-based ones) can offer relief. It's important to consult with your doctor to determine what medications, if any, are best suited for your condition.

- **Heat and Cold Therapy**: The use of **cold packs** for inflammation or swelling and **heat pads** for muscle relaxation is often a first-line therapy. You can even combine both methods—alternating between heat and cold to help with various types of pain. **Cold therapy** is particularly effective in the first 24-48 hours after an injury, while **heat therapy** can help relax stiff muscles or alleviate chronic pain.

- **Topical Creams and Gels**: For localized pain, especially in conditions like arthritis or muscle strains, topical analgesics like **lidocaine** or **menthol-based gels** can offer temporary relief without the side effects associated with oral medications.

- **TENS Units** (Transcutaneous Electrical Nerve Stimulation): A portable, non-invasive device that sends electrical impulses through the skin to block pain signals. It's used in conditions such as **back pain** and **osteoarthritis** and can provide short-term relief.

- **Mindfulness and Breathing Techniques**: When pain is overwhelming, techniques like **deep breathing**, **progressive muscle relaxation**, or **guided meditation** can quickly shift your focus away from pain. This doesn't eliminate the pain, but it helps to reduce its perception and provides mental relief.

3. Long-Term Management: Building Lasting Relief

While immediate relief is important, the goal of pain management is to build a system that provides long-term relief. This is where we begin incorporating **lifestyle adjustments**, **exercise**, and **dietary changes** into your toolkit.

- **Physical Therapy**: A physical therapist can help design an **exercise program** tailored to your condition. For example, if you suffer from **chronic lower back pain**, specific exercises can strengthen the muscles around the spine, improving support and decreasing discomfort. Regular **stretching routines** can improve flexibility and reduce pain from stiff joints or muscles.
- **Strengthening Exercises**: For those with **joint pain**, strengthening the muscles around the affected joint can provide better support and reduce pressure on the bones and tissues. This is particularly important for those with conditions like **osteoarthritis**.
- **Yoga and Pilates**: Both are excellent for improving flexibility, core strength, and posture—key factors in managing chronic pain. Yoga's focus on mindful movement and breath can be particularly beneficial for managing pain related to **stress** or **tension**.

- **Ergonomic Adjustments**: Pay attention to how your body interacts with your environment. Is your desk or workstation set up in a way that promotes proper posture? Are you using tools or furniture that help alleviate strain? Small ergonomic changes can make a huge difference in long-term pain relief, particularly for those suffering from repetitive strain injuries or neck and back pain.

- **Diet and Nutrition**: As mentioned earlier, food can play a major role in pain management. A diet rich in **anti-inflammatory foods** like **omega-3 fatty acids**, **leafy greens**, and **berries** can help reduce inflammation in the body. For individuals with **gut-related issues**, foods that promote a healthy gut microbiome may also play a role in reducing pain.

4. Psychological Tools: Addressing the Mind-Body Connection

Since pain is not just a physical experience but also a **psychological** one, it's important to include **mental health strategies** in your toolkit. Chronic pain can take a significant emotional toll, and managing the emotional aspects is just as crucial as addressing the physical ones.

- **Cognitive Behavioral Therapy (CBT)**: CBT is a well-researched therapy that helps individuals with chronic pain by teaching them to identify negative thought patterns that can worsen the pain experience. It helps individuals change their perceptions of pain and manage emotions like frustration, anger, and fear.

- **Mindfulness-Based Stress Reduction (MBSR)**: This technique teaches you to focus on the present moment without judgment, which can greatly reduce the emotional response to pain. MBSR has been shown to improve pain tolerance and reduce pain-related stress.
- **Support Groups**: Chronic pain can feel isolating, but connecting with others who are going through similar experiences can be incredibly therapeutic. Support groups provide emotional validation and a safe space to share coping strategies.

5. Tracking Progress and Making Adjustments

A key component of your pain management toolkit is **tracking your progress**. This means regularly monitoring your pain levels, triggers, and responses to the tools and strategies you've implemented. Keep a **pain journal**, noting down how different activities, foods, medications, and therapies impact your pain. This will allow us to adjust your plan over time, ensuring that your toolkit remains effective and aligned with your evolving needs.

Conclusion: A Toolkit That Works for You

Your pain management toolkit is not static. It's a living, breathing system that will evolve over time, shaped by your personal experiences and preferences. The goal is to equip you with a range of strategies that give you the **freedom** to manage your pain and reclaim your life. Remember, it's not about curing pain completely—it's about finding ways to **live well** despite it.

Together, we can customize a toolkit that fits **your life**, **your pain**, and **your goals**—one that empowers you to make informed decisions and actively manage your pain. The more tools you have, the more confident you'll feel in your tailored pain management.

7.4 Personalized Pain Strategies: Where to Begin

When it comes to managing pain, **one size does not fit all**. Each person experiences pain differently, and what works for one person might not work for another. As a doctor, my primary goal is to guide you toward a **personalized pain strategy** that is tailored specifically to **your needs**, **your condition**, and **your lifestyle**. A personalized strategy allows us to take a more holistic approach to managing your pain, addressing not just the physical symptoms but also the emotional and mental aspects of your pain journey.

Step 1: Understanding Your Pain

The foundation of any personalized pain strategy starts with a **comprehensive understanding** of your pain. We need to ask key questions such as:

- **Where is the pain?** Is it localized or widespread?
- **What type of pain are you experiencing?** Is it sharp, dull, aching, burning, or throbbing?
- **When does it occur?** Is it constant, or does it come and go?
- **What triggers the pain?** Are there specific activities, foods, or emotions that make it worse?

- **What helps relieve the pain?** Do certain movements, medications, or treatments bring some relief?

This information will form the basis of your strategy. Identifying the **root causes** of your pain, as well as its **patterns**, helps us understand the best approach to take.

Step 2: Collaborating on Your Treatment Goals

Once we have a clear understanding of your pain, the next step is to **define your treatment goals**. These goals should be specific, measurable, and **realistic**. It's essential that these goals align with your overall lifestyle and health aspirations. For example:

- Are you looking for immediate pain relief or long-term management?
- Do you want to focus on reducing medication use, or are you comfortable integrating medications into your plan?
- Are you seeking a more active approach, such as physical therapy or exercise?
- Do you prefer to address pain through natural remedies, or are you open to more traditional medical interventions?

Having these clear goals ensures that we can develop a plan that works specifically for you, allowing you to feel confident in your approach.

Step 3: Selecting the Right Tools for Your Toolkit

After we've clarified your goals, it's time to choose the right combination of **treatments and tools** for your pain management toolkit. This might include:

1. **Medications**: Depending on your pain's intensity and type, we might recommend prescription pain relievers, over-the-counter medication, or topical analgesics. It's important to use these carefully and in conjunction with other methods to avoid becoming overly reliant on them.
2. **Physical Therapy**: A well-structured physical therapy program is often key to managing pain, particularly for **joint and musculoskeletal conditions**. It can help strengthen muscles, improve flexibility, and reduce strain on affected areas. I may recommend specific exercises designed to **target** your pain areas and improve overall mobility.
3. **Mind-Body Techniques**: Since pain is both a physical and emotional experience, techniques like **mindfulness**, **deep breathing**, and **meditation** can help reduce the **emotional distress** that often accompanies pain. Regular practice of these techniques can improve your overall sense of well-being and make pain feel more manageable.
4. **Nutritional Support**: Diet plays a huge role in managing pain, especially for inflammatory conditions. I may suggest incorporating **anti-inflammatory foods** like omega-3-rich fish, **turmeric**, and **leafy greens** into your meals. I may

also recommend supplements such as **vitamin D**, **magnesium**, or **glucosamine** to support joint health and reduce inflammation.

5. **Alternative Therapies**: In some cases, non-traditional therapies like **acupuncture**, **massage**, or **chiropractic care** can provide relief for certain types of pain. These therapies often help by improving blood flow, relieving muscle tension, and stimulating the body's natural healing processes.
6. **Technology-Assisted Therapies**: Depending on your condition, I may also suggest innovative treatments such as **TENS** (transcutaneous electrical nerve stimulation), **virtual reality therapy**, or other advanced technologies that help manage pain in a non-invasive way.

Step 4: Implementing Lifestyle Adjustments

Personalized pain management also requires making adjustments to your **lifestyle**. The way you move, rest, eat, and even think can significantly impact your pain levels. Small changes can lead to big improvements in how you feel. This might include:

- **Posture and Ergonomics**: If your pain is related to repetitive strain or poor posture (e.g., back or neck pain), we will work together on setting up your workspace, improving your posture, and incorporating regular movement breaks into your routine.
- **Exercise and Physical Activity**: Regular physical activity is crucial for long-term pain management. I

will help you find an exercise program that works with your condition. This may include **low-impact activities** like swimming, walking, or yoga, which can help keep you mobile and reduce stiffness.

- **Sleep Hygiene**: Poor sleep can worsen pain, so I'll provide tips on improving your sleep environment and habits. Ensuring you get enough restorative sleep is key to managing both the **physical** and **mental** aspects of pain.

- **Stress Management**: Chronic stress can make pain worse. Developing **stress management** strategies such as **journaling**, **hobbies**, or spending time with loved ones can help lower stress hormones that can exacerbate pain.

Step 5: Regular Monitoring and Adjustments

A personalized pain strategy is **not static**. It requires **regular monitoring** and adjustments based on your progress. Together, we will track your pain levels, the effectiveness of different strategies, and any changes you notice in your symptoms.

- **Keep a Pain Journal**: Document your pain experiences, including triggers, treatments, and relief methods. This can help us understand what works and what doesn't, and refine your approach over time.

- **Stay Open to Changes**: As your condition evolves, so will your pain management plan. Be open to trying new treatments or adjusting existing ones as necessary. Sometimes, what works at one stage may need to be replaced or combined with other strategies later on.

Step 6: Collaboration and Support

Your pain management strategy is a **team effort**. It's important to communicate openly with me, your family, and other healthcare professionals. Whether it's asking about a new therapy, discussing side effects of medications, or addressing concerns with a new lifestyle change, **ongoing dialogue** is crucial for achieving the best outcomes.

- **Family Involvement**: Having the support of your loved ones can significantly impact your ability to manage pain. I'll encourage family members to learn about your pain and how they can help.
- **Second Opinions**: If you feel that your strategy is not yielding the desired results, or if you want additional perspectives, don't hesitate to seek a second opinion. I'll guide you through this process to ensure that you're getting the best care possible.

Conclusion: A Personalized Approach to a Better Life

Creating a personalized pain management strategy is not just about managing pain; it's about **reclaiming your life**. By understanding your pain, setting realistic goals, and incorporating the right tools and strategies, you will have the power to not only manage it but thrive despite it.

Remember, your strategy is unique to you. It's about finding what works best for your body, your condition, and your goals. Together, we will navigate this journey, adjusting and refining your plan as needed to help you live your life with as little pain and as much vitality as possible.

7.5 From Patient to Advocate: Sharing Your Pain Story

As you navigate your pain journey, it's straightforward to feel isolated, misunderstood, or even helpless at times. But over the years, I have seen a profound shift in how patients can take charge of their experience and transform from individuals suffering in silence into empowered advocates. Sharing your pain story not only provides relief for yourself, but also serves as a platform for others who may share your feelings but lack the courage or voice to voice them.

The Healing Power of Sharing Your Story

Sharing your pain story is often a **healing act**. It gives you the opportunity to reflect on your journey, process your emotions, and come to terms with your experiences. It also allows you to **connect with others** who are going through similar challenges. This connection can lead to a powerful sense of community, solidarity, and **understanding** — something many people with chronic pain feel they lack.

I encourage you to think of your pain story as a **tool for healing**, not just for yourself, yourself but for others who may find strength in your words. When you share your experience, you give voice to something that many people feel but often can't articulate. **Your story is valid, and it matters**.

Why Advocacy Matters

Advocacy begins when you decide to take your pain and turn it into **action**. By sharing your pain story, you have the potential to raise awareness about the invisible struggles of living with chronic pain, **educate others**, and encourage those in pain to seek help.

1. **Raising Awareness**: Many people still misunderstand or dismiss chronic pain, thinking of it as something minor or temporary. By speaking up, you can change this narrative. **Raising awareness** is crucial for improving public understanding and healthcare resources dedicated to pain management.

2. **Advocating for Better Care**: Sharing your experience is also an essential step in pushing for better medical care. Many healthcare systems still fail to prioritize pain management adequately, leaving patients without proper treatments or support. **Your voice** can help push for better policies, better research, and better care options for others.

3. **Fighting the Stigma**: Chronic pain often carries a stigma that causes many people to suffer in silence. They fear being labeled as weak, lazy, or dramatic. But the truth is, chronic pain is real, and it affects millions of people. By sharing your story, you help **normalize the conversation** about pain and encourage others to stop hiding it.

4. **Empowering Others**: There are countless individuals who are suffering in silence, unsure where to turn for help. Your story might be the beacon of hope someone else needs to find their voice or take their first step toward treatment. When you share, you create a ripple effect that empowers others to speak up and ask for the help they deserve.

How to Become an Advocate

Turning from a patient into an advocate doesn't have to be overwhelming. It can start with small, meaningful actions:

1. **Sharing Your Story Locally**: Start by sharing your experience with family, friends, or support groups. This helps build a foundation of empathy and understanding, making it easier to advocate for your own needs in the future.
2. **Engaging on Social Media**: Platforms like Instagram, Twitter, or even blog posts can give you a voice in the wider community. Use these platforms to educate others about the realities of chronic pain, share your personal struggles, and offer support to others who are going through similar experiences.
3. **Joining Advocacy Groups**: There are many organizations and online communities dedicated to chronic pain awareness and advocacy. These groups are filled with people who share your experiences and goals. Becoming involved in these communities can amplify your voice and connect you with others who are passionate about the same issues.

4. **Speaking Out in Your Doctor's Office**: Never underestimate the power of speaking up during your medical appointments. Use your voice to ask questions, raise concerns, and ensure your treatment is aligned with your needs. A great advocate for your own health is a **well-informed patient** who isn't afraid to express what they're feeling and ask for the best care possible.
5. **Becoming a Resource**: As you gather more knowledge about your pain condition and the treatments available, you can become a resource for others. Offering advice or sharing your coping strategies can make a huge difference to someone who is just beginning their journey with pain.

Turning Advocacy into Action

If you feel passionate about making a lasting difference in the world of chronic pain management, your advocacy can extend into **action**. You may want to consider:

- **Lobbying for Policy Changes**: There are many patient advocacy groups that work tirelessly to push for better policies, funding for research, and healthcare reforms. By joining these movements, you can be part of the larger push to change how chronic pain is understood and treated at a national or global level.
- **Supporting Pain Research**: Contributing to or supporting pain research organizations is another way to make a significant impact. The more we understand about pain, the better equipped we are to

treat it effectively. Supporting research can give future generations of pain patients better options and hope for lasting relief.

- **Educating Healthcare Providers**: Some doctors may not fully understand the complexities of pain, especially when it's not visible. By sharing your story with your healthcare providers or offering to participate in training sessions for new medical professionals, you can help ensure that future patients are treated with empathy and expertise.

The Impact of Advocacy on You

While sharing your story can make a huge difference for others, it can also benefit you in profound ways. Advocacy helps shift the focus from your own suffering to something that is larger than yourself. **By helping others, you gain a sense of purpose**, which can be incredibly powerful when coping with chronic pain. Advocacy also reinforces your **sense of agency**—you are no longer just a passive recipient of treatment, treatment but an active participant in improving not only your own life but the lives of others as well.

Conclusion: Your Voice Matters

You are not just a patient; you are a **storyteller**, a **voice of experience**, and a **warrior**. Every story shared, every conversation started, and every bit of awareness raised brings us one step closer to a world that truly understands chronic pain. Your pain does not define you, but how you respond to it and advocate for others can create ripples of change that last far beyond your individual journey.

Remember, **your pain story matters**. It's a vital part of the narrative that can transform lives, including your own. By sharing your story, you help yourself and many others who feel invisible or unheard. Let your voice echo — it has the power to inspire, heal, and create real change.

Chapter - 8

Navigating The System For Relief

8.1 Choosing the Right Specialist

As someone who has spent years treating patients, I understand how overwhelming it can be to navigate the complex world of pain management. The road to relief often involves seeing multiple specialists, trying various treatments, and making countless decisions. But the first, and most crucial, step in this journey is choosing the right specialist.

Selecting the right doctor or pain management specialist can significantly impact your recovery. It's not just about finding someone with the appropriate qualifications or experience, but also someone who aligns with your personal needs and values. Let me guide you through this process, which can often feel like an intimidating maze.

Understanding the Different Types of Specialists

Pain management is an intricate field that requires expertise across various disciplines. Depending on the type and source of your pain, you may be referred to different specialists. Here are a few of the most common:

1. **Pain Management Specialists**: These are doctors specifically trained to treat all types of pain, including chronic pain, neuropathic pain, and musculoskeletal pain. They typically have expertise in various treatment methods, including medication management, nerve blocks, and minimally invasive procedures. They are a great option if your pain has persisted for a long time and other treatments haven't worked.

2. **Orthopedic Surgeons**: If your pain is musculoskeletal, especially related to bones, joints, or muscles, an orthopedic surgeon can evaluate your condition. They can help with conditions like arthritis, tendon injuries, and spinal issues. Some orthopedic surgeons specialize in specific areas, like the knee or spine, so be sure to find someone with expertise in your particular area of concern.

3. **Neurologists**: Neurologists focus on pain caused by nerve damage or dysfunction. If you are experiencing neuropathic pain, such as tingling, burning, or shooting pains, this may be the right specialist for you. They are particularly skilled in diagnosing and treating conditions like sciatica, diabetic neuropathy, or post-surgical pain.

4. **Rheumatologists**: These doctors specialize in autoimmune conditions and inflammatory diseases that affect the joints, such as rheumatoid arthritis, lupus, and ankylosing spondylitis. If your pain is due

to chronic inflammation, a rheumatologist's expertise will be invaluable.

5. **Physiotherapists**: While not medical doctors, physiotherapists play a crucial role in pain management. They use physical therapy techniques such as manual therapy, exercise, and modalities like heat and cold therapy to improve mobility, reduce pain, and strengthen the muscles and joints. A physiotherapist can be a key part of your overall treatment plan, especially if you are recovering from an injury or surgery.

6. **Psychologists or Psychiatrists**: Chronic pain often has a psychological component, and mental health professionals can be an integral part of your healing process. They can help you manage the emotional impact of pain, address stress, anxiety, or depression, and provide techniques like cognitive behavioral therapy (CBT) that have been shown to be effective in managing chronic pain.

What to Look for in a Specialist

Now that you understand the types of specialists you might encounter, let's talk about what you should look for when selecting the right one for your pain management journey:

1. **Experience and Expertise**: It's important to choose a specialist who has experience treating the specific type of pain you are experiencing. Ask about their training, credentials, and track record with patients who have similar conditions. It's crucial to feel confident in their expertise and approach.

2. **Holistic Approach**: Pain management is not just about prescribing medications or performing surgery. Look for specialists who take a **holistic** approach, considering not just the physical aspects of your pain, but also the emotional, psychological, and lifestyle factors that may be contributing to your condition. A specialist who understands the full picture can offer more comprehensive and lasting solutions.

3. **Communication Style**: A key part of any treatment plan is a trusting relationship with your doctor. You should feel comfortable discussing your symptoms, asking questions, and expressing concerns. Choose a specialist who listens attentively, explains your condition clearly, and involves you in decision-making. Clear communication fosters trust and can make all the difference in your treatment experience.

4. **Approach to Pain Management**: Some specialists may rely heavily on medications, while others may emphasize physical therapy or non-invasive treatments first. Depending on your preferences and values, you may want to find someone who aligns with your approach to treatment. For example, if you are hesitant about surgery, you might prefer a specialist who focuses on non-surgical options.

5. **Reputation and Reviews**: While this isn't everything, a specialist's reputation can be a good indicator of the quality of care you can expect. Look for patient reviews or testimonials. You can also ask your primary care doctor or friends and family for

recommendations. **Word of mouth** can often lead you to a compassionate and effective provider.

Questions to Ask During Your First Appointment

Once you've narrowed down your options, it's time to meet with the specialist. Here are some questions that can help you assess whether this is the right fit for you:

- What is your approach to treating chronic pain, and how do you customize treatments for individual patients?
- What are my treatment options, and what are their potential side effects or risks?
- How do you work with other healthcare providers, such as physiotherapists or psychologists, to create a comprehensive pain management plan?
- Are you open to non-medication-based treatments like physical therapy, acupuncture, or cognitive behavioral therapy?
- How do you track progress and adjust treatments over time?
- How will you help me manage any emotional or psychological challenges related to chronic pain?

Remember, choosing the right specialist is not a one-time decision. It's okay to seek a second opinion or try a different doctor if you feel that your needs aren't being met. **Advocacy for your own health** is about finding the right fit, fit—someone who respects your concerns and is committed to helping you manage your pain in the best possible way.

Conclusion: You Deserve the Best Care

The journey toward pain relief is not always straightforward, but with the right specialist by your side, you can feel empowered. Take your time, ask the right questions, and be your own advocate. When you find the right specialist, they will guide you through pain relief with expertise, compassion, and a commitment to your needs.

Choosing the right specialist can be one of the most important decisions you make in your pain management journey. Take your time, do your research, and remember: You deserve to have a partner in this journey who listens, understands, and works with you to achieve the best possible outcome.

8.2 How to Interpret Medical Advice

As a patient, interpreting medical advice can often feel like deciphering a complex language. Doctors and specialists are trained to think critically and provide detailed information, but it's common for patients to leave a consultation feeling uncertain, overwhelmed, or unsure about how to proceed. As someone who has spent years guiding patients through the complexities of pain management, I understand the importance of not just hearing medical advice, advice but truly understanding and making sense of it in the context of your life.

In this section, I'll walk you through how to interpret medical advice effectively, ensuring you feel empowered to make informed decisions about your treatment plan.

1. Understand the Terminology

One of the biggest challenges in interpreting medical advice is understanding the jargon used by healthcare providers. Words like "neuropathic," "degenerative," or "biopsy" may sound foreign, but understanding these terms is essential in making informed decisions about your care.

Here are a few tips to help with this:

- **Don't be afraid to ask questions**: If a term or procedure is unclear, ask the doctor to explain it in simpler terms. A good doctor will want to ensure you understand the information.
- **Research**: While you should never substitute online research for professional medical advice, doing a little research on terms that confuse you can help you better understand your diagnosis. Trust reputable sources, like medical journals or well-established health organizations.
- **Use diagrams or written materials**: Ask your doctor if they have brochures, diagrams, or websites they recommend to help you better understand your condition. Some doctors may even offer a follow-up appointment to address questions after you've had time to absorb the information.

2. Clarify the Rationale Behind the Recommendation

Medical advice often comes with a specific recommendation: a test, a treatment, a medication, or even a lifestyle change. However, it's crucial to comprehend the rationale behind this advice.

Ask your doctor:

- **What is the goal of this treatment?** Understand what the treatment is meant to achieve. Is it pain relief, increased mobility, or the prevention of further complications?
- **What are the risks and benefits?** Every treatment comes with its potential advantages and drawbacks. Your doctor should be able to clearly outline both. This will help you weigh the options and make an informed decision.
- **How does this fit into my overall treatment plan?** Ask how the advice or treatment fits within the context of your broader pain management strategy. If it's part of a multi-faceted approach, understanding how everything works together will give you confidence in the treatment process.

Understanding the rationale helps you take ownership of your treatment plan and gives you confidence in your choices.

3. Recognize Your Own Values and Preferences

Medical advice should be based on both the doctor's expertise and your values and preferences. You are the one living with pain and managing your treatment, so your thoughts, concerns, and preferences should always be considered.

- **Lifestyle considerations**: Consider how the recommended treatment will impact your daily life. Will it require significant changes to your routine? Is it feasible given your lifestyle and commitments?
- **Personal goals**: If your goal is to avoid surgery at all costs, this is important to communicate to your doctor. Similarly, if you're interested in exploring non-medication-based treatments, make sure your doctor is aware of your preferences.
- **Quality of life**: Some treatments may reduce pain but come with side effects that diminish your overall quality of life. It's important to weigh these factors and prioritize your long-term well-being.

Understanding your own values can help you filter medical advice through the lens of what truly matters to you.

4. Consider Second Opinions and Ask for Clarification

It's completely acceptable, and often advisable, to seek a second opinion, especially if you're uncertain about a diagnosis or treatment plan. A second opinion can offer reassurance or alternative solutions that you might not have been aware of.

When you seek a second opinion, it's important to:to

- **Bring your medical records**: Make sure you have a full record of your diagnosis, previous treatments, and any tests or imaging results. This will help the second doctor assess your situation accurately.

- **Ask the same questions**: When meeting with the second specialist, ask the same questions you asked your first doctor to ensure you're comparing the information equally.
- **Trust your instincts**: While a second opinion is valuable, trust your own judgment in interpreting the advice. If something feels off or doesn't align with your values, it's important to advocate for yourself and explore your options further.

5. Follow Up and Track Progress

Medical advice is not a one-time event. As treatment progresses, it's important to follow up with your healthcare provider to track your progress, assess the effectiveness of the treatment, and address any new symptoms or concerns.

- **Be proactive about follow-ups**: Make sure you have follow-up appointments scheduled, especially if your treatment involves medication changes, physical therapy, or a new lifestyle plan.
- **Keep a pain diary**: Document your symptoms, medication usage, side effects, and other relevant information to discuss with your doctor at follow-ups. This helps both you and your doctor evaluate the treatment's success and make any necessary adjustments.
- **Ask for clarification when needed**: If something changes in your condition or if you're unsure about

the next steps, don't hesitate to reach out to your healthcare provider for further clarification.

6. Understand the Role of Self-Advocacy

While doctors provide guidance, ultimately, you are the best advocate for your own health. Medical advice should empower you to take control of your pain management. If a doctor's advice feels unclear or misaligned with your needs, it's okay to ask for clarification, request alternatives, or even explore a new provider. Remember that this is your body, and your doctor is there to help guide you—not dictate your choices.

Advocacy is not just about asking questions; it's about actively engaging in your care. Make sure to:

- **Ask about alternatives**: If you're uncomfortable with a particular treatment, ask your doctor if there are other options available.
- **Understand your role**: Treatment is often a partnership. Know that your own efforts—whether through lifestyle changes, physical therapy, or emotional support—play a significant role in your recovery.
- **Empower yourself**: Empowerment comes from understanding your condition and the treatments available to you. The more informed you are, the better equipped you'll be to make decisions that align with your health goals.

Conclusion: Take Charge of Your Pain Journey

Interpreting medical advice is not just about understanding the words; it's about understanding *how those words affect you.* It's about taking ownership of your health and ensuring that the advice you receive is the best for your unique situation.

I encourage you to ask questions, seek clarity, and be proactive in your treatment decisions. Your healthcare providers will guide you, but you know your body best. When you understand medical advice, you are better equipped to control your pain journey and work with your healthcare team toward the relief and well-being you deserve.

8.3 The Role of Caregivers in Pain Management

As a doctor who frequently works with patients suffering from chronic pain, I cannot stress enough the crucial role caregivers play in the journey toward pain relief and management. While medical interventions are essential, caregivers provide the everyday support that often makes the biggest difference in a patient's quality of life. This chapter will explore the vital role caregivers play in pain management, the emotional and physical demands they face, and how they can better support those in pain.

1. The Emotional Support System

Pain—especially chronic pain—can feel isolating. It's not just the physical discomfort, but the emotional toll it takes on patients, leaving them feeling frustrated, hopeless, or even depressed. This is where caregivers step in. They are often the ones who bear witness to the patient's struggles, offering comfort, encouragement, and a sense of security. Emotional support plays a significant role in pain management; patients who feel emotionally supported are often better equipped to manage their pain.

Caregivers can provide emotional support by:

- **Listening without judgment**: Sometimes, patients just need someone who will listen to them. Simply being there to hear their frustrations or fears can provide significant relief.
- **Offering encouragement**: Chronic pain can make even the simplest tasks seem impossible. Caregivers can help by encouraging patients to continue with their treatment plans, maintain mobility, and not give up on their recovery.
- **Maintaining a positive outlook**: While it's important to validate a patient's feelings, caregivers can also help by encouraging optimism. Reminding patients that they are not alone in their journey toward pain relief can offer a much-needed sense of hope.

2. Practical Assistance with Daily Tasks

Chronic pain often impacts a patient's ability to carry out daily activities. Whether it's managing household chores, preparing meals, or even personal care tasks, pain can make these activities feel overwhelming. A caregiver's role here is multifaceted—helping patients maintain as much independence as possible while providing support when Instagram reel necessary.

Caregivers assist by:

- **Assisting with mobility**: Some patients with chronic pain struggle with movement, which can affect their ability to walk, climb stairs, or even stand for long periods. Caregivers may help with mobility aids, assist in physical therapy exercises, or provide physical support in getting from one place to another.
- **Helping with personal care**: Basic tasks such as bathing, dressing, or grooming can become challenging for those in chronic pain. Caregivers offer assistance with these tasks while also respecting the patient's dignity and sense of independence.
- **Managing daily routines**: A caregiver can help ensure that patients take their medications on time, follow their prescribed exercise regimens, and adhere to any other aspects of their treatment plan.

3. Monitoring Symptoms and Treatment Adherence

For a patient with chronic pain, monitoring symptoms and adhering to treatment plans can become difficult due to mental fatigue or physical limitations. Caregivers can help patients stay on track by closely observing changes in symptoms, ensuring that prescribed treatments are followed, and noting any side effects or improvements.

Here’s how caregivers can assist in this role:

- **Tracking progress**: Keep a log of the patient's symptoms, treatments, and any changes that occur over time. This can help both the patient and doctor assess the effectiveness of a treatment plan and make necessary adjustments.

- **Prompting medication adherence**: Many pain management plans involve complex medication schedules. Caregivers can help by reminding the patient to take their medications as prescribed and ensuring they are taken correctly.
- **Reporting changes to healthcare providers**: If there is a noticeable improvement or deterioration in the patient's condition, caregivers can communicate these changes to the doctor. This feedback can guide adjustments to treatment plans.

4. Navigating the Emotional and Physical Stress of Caregiving

The role of a caregiver can be physically and emotionally taxing. While providing care to a loved one or patient, caregivers often experience stress, anxiety, and burnout. It's essential for caregivers to take care of themselves so that they can continue providing effective support to their loved ones.

Caregivers can prevent burnout by:

- **Taking regular breaks**: Caregiving can be overwhelming, and caregivers often forget to take time for themselves. Whether it's a short walk, a hobby, or a day off, caregivers must find time to recharge.
- **Seeking support**: Caregivers should not feel they have to do everything on their own. Reaching out for

support—whether through family members, friends, or caregiver support groups—can help relieve stress.

- **Learning to ask for help**: Caregivers may hesitate to ask for help out of a sense of duty or guilt. However, recognizing when extra assistance is needed—whether it's from professional home care providers or family members—can prevent caregivers from burning out.

5. Educating and Empowering Caregivers

Effective pain management goes beyond just medication and physical treatment. Educating caregivers about pain, its effects, and available treatments is vital. When caregivers are educated, they are better equipped to provide the appropriate support and understand what their loved ones are going through.

Caregivers can benefit from:

- **Learning about the condition**: The more caregivers understand about the patient's specific pain condition—whether it's arthritis, neuropathic pain, or something else—the better they can assist in managing symptoms.
- **Understanding pain management techniques**: Caregivers should learn about different pain management strategies, such as relaxation exercises, deep breathing, or gentle massage, that can complement medical treatments.
- **Knowing when to seek medical help**: While caregivers can manage day-to-day care, it's essential for them to know when symptoms worsen or when

something seems off. Being educated about when to call the doctor can make all the difference in preventing complications.

6. The Importance of Communication Between Caregivers and Healthcare Providers

Clear and open communication between caregivers and healthcare providers is a cornerstone of effective pain management. Caregivers are often the primary source of information about a patient's daily condition, and doctors rely on them to provide updates and feedback.

Caregivers can facilitate this communication by:

- **Sharing observations**: By keeping the healthcare provider informed of any changes in the patient's condition, caregivers help doctors fine-tune treatments and adjust care plans accordingly.
- **Being an advocate for the patient**: Caregivers can advocate for their loved one by ensuring that their pain management needs are addressed, that they are being heard, and that all aspects of their health are taken into consideration.
- **Building a collaborative relationship**: Establishing a strong relationship with the healthcare team allows caregivers to be more involved in decision-making processes and ensure that they're equipped to help manage the patient's care.

Conclusion: A Crucial Part of the Healing Journey

One cannot overstate the importance of caregivers in pain management. They provide emotional support, physical assistance, and vital monitoring of the treatment process. Caregivers often face significant challenges, both emotionally and physically, but their dedication plays an indispensable role in helping patients manage their pain. By educating and supporting caregivers, we can create a more holistic and compassionate approach to pain management that empowers both patients and their loved ones.

As a doctor, I encourage caregivers to not only focus on their loved one's needs but to take care of their own well-being as well. When both the patient and the caregiver are supported, the journey toward pain relief becomes a shared experience—one that offers the best chance for healing and a better quality of life.

8.4 Fighting for Insurance Coverage

In my practice, I often witness patients struggling to secure insurance coverage for essential pain treatments, which is a significant source of frustration. As a doctor, I've seen how crucial it is for patients to have access to the right care, yet many are held back by bureaucratic red tape and insurance limitations. Navigating the world of insurance coverage for pain management is not only challenging but can also feel discouraging for patients and their families. This chapter will focus on understanding the insurance landscape, how to advocate for the treatments your patients need, and the steps you can take to ensure the best outcomes in the face of insurance roadblocks.

1. The Challenges of Insurance Coverage for Pain Treatment

Pain is a complex condition—what works for one person may not work for another. Unfortunately, insurance companies often operate on rigid guidelines that don't always reflect the unique needs of patients. These policies can be a barrier to receiving appropriate and timely treatments. Common obstacles include:

- **Restricted treatment options**: Many insurance companies have a limited range of treatments they cover, often favoring short-term solutions like painkillers, while more holistic or advanced therapies, such as physical therapy, acupuncture, or nerve blocks, may not be covered.
- **Pre-authorization requirements**: A significant barrier is the need for pre-authorization, where insurance companies require approval before a treatment can be started. This process can delay the care a patient urgently needs.
- **Denial of coverage**: In some cases, the insurance provider denies coverage altogether, citing that the treatment is not medically necessary or that it falls outside the scope of their policies.

The urgency and frustration of dealing with ongoing pain often compound these challenges for patients. For caregivers and healthcare professionals, the added stress of navigating insurance systems can feel overwhelming.

2. Understanding Insurance Policies and Limits

It's essential to understand the specifics of a patient's insurance coverage before initiating treatment plans. Every insurance policy has its own terms, and a treatment plan that is covered by one provider may not be covered by another. As a healthcare provider, you should be well-versed in the details of the insurance plans your patients hold so you can anticipate potential roadblocks.

- **Know the formulary**: Insurance companies often maintain a formulary, a list of medications and treatments they approve. It's important to familiarize yourself with the formulary to guide your patients toward options that are more likely to be approved.

- **Understand exclusions**: Policies may have exclusions for certain treatments or conditions. Review these exclusions closely to ensure that you're recommending options that have the best chance of being covered.

- **Advocate for medically necessary treatments**: Sometimes, insurance companies may deny coverage based on the treatment being deemed "experimental" or "non-essential." However, as a doctor, you can fight for medically necessary treatments by providing clear documentation of their importance in the patient's health journey.

3. Steps for Patients and Healthcare Providers to Take

If a patient's insurance refuses to cover a treatment or therapy you deem essential, it doesn't mean the end of the journey.

There are several proactive steps both patients and providers can take to fight for the care they deserve:

- **Appealing the denial**: Insurers often give patients the option to appeal denials. As a healthcare provider, you can help by drafting letters of medical necessity, providing detailed documentation about why a specific treatment is required, and detailing the patient's history of unsuccessful treatments.
- **Providing medical evidence**: Insurers may need concrete evidence to reconsider a denial. You can help by submitting comprehensive documentation that supports the need for the treatment, such as clinical studies, expert opinions, and a history of the patient's previous treatment failures.
- **Exploring alternative treatments**: If a particular treatment is denied, it may be helpful to explore alternatives that could be covered under the policy. This may involve adjusting your treatment plan, but it can still provide relief while the insurance company reviews the initial request.
- **Working with insurance advocates**: Some healthcare providers or patients may benefit from insurance advocacy services, either through a lawyer, patient advocacy group, or a specialized

insurance professional who can help navigate the process. These experts can assist with appeals and understand the intricacies of insurance policies.

4. **Collaboration with Patients to Understand Their Options**

It's crucial to keep patients informed throughout the insurance process. For many patients, the issue of insurance can feel like an additional weight on top of their physical pain. As a doctor, your role in supporting them is multifaceted:multifaceted.

- **Empower patients to ask questions**: Encourage your patients to be proactive about their insurance coverage. Help them understand the nuances of their policies, and guide them on how to ask the right questions when contacting insurance companies.
- **Help with paperwork**: Navigating insurance policies often involves a lot of paperwork, which can be time-consuming and confusing. As part of the care process, guide patients through the necessary steps and forms, ensuring they have everything needed for appeals or additional requests.
- **Emotional support**: Dealing with insurance can add a layer of emotional stress for patients already dealing with chronic pain. Offering a supportive, empathetic presence can help patients feel less overwhelmed during these challenging times.

5. Advocating for Systemic Change

Beyond the individual patient's fight for coverage, there is a need for systemic change. The current state of insurance coverage for pain treatments is inadequate and often out of touch with patients' realities. As healthcare providers, it is our responsibility to advocate for broader change that makes pain management more accessible.

- **Collaborate with patient advocacy groups**: There are numerous organizations dedicated to improving insurance coverage for pain management. By supporting these organizations or becoming involved in advocacy efforts, you can help bring about the changes needed to provide better care for patients.
- **Raise awareness**: Talk to policymakers, write to insurance companies, and support initiatives that push for broader coverage for pain treatments. By joining forces with others in the medical community and patient groups, you can help amplify the voices of those who suffer from chronic pain.

6. The Bottom Line: Persistence Pays Off

Fighting for insurance coverage can be exhausting and frustrating, but it is crucial in ensuring that patients receive the care they need. As doctors, our advocacy for our patients doesn't end with the treatment we provide—it extends to ensuring that they have access to that treatment. By helping patients navigate the insurance process, being proactive in appeals, and pushing for systemic change, we can pave the way for a more supportive and accessible pain management landscape.

The battle with insurance is not easy, but it is worth the effort. Every patient deserves the right to effective treatment, and with persistence, advocacy, and collaboration, we can help ensure they get it.

Chapter - 9
Rethinking Pain Through Innovation

9.1 Wearable Technology for Chronic Pain Monitoring

As a pain specialist, I've witnessed the remarkable strides we've made in understanding and managing chronic pain, but we still face significant challenges. One of the most persistent issues with chronic pain is the difficulty in accurately monitoring it. Pain, afterAfter all, all, pain is subjective—what one person experiences as a 6/10 may feel completely different to another person. And for many of my patients, their pain fluctuates over time, making it challenging to track progress or detect patterns.

This is where wearable technology can play a transformative role.

In recent years, advancements in wearable devices have begun to offer us a more precise, real-time way of monitoring pain. As a doctor, I've seen firsthand how these innovations are changing the way we approach pain management. These devices are no longer a futuristic idea; they are here and now, becoming powerful tools in the fight against chronic pain.

How Wearable Technology Works for Chronic Pain Monitoring

At the core of wearable technology for pain management is the ability to continuously track a patient's physiological responses, often in ways that were previously not possible. Whether through sensors that measure heart rate, skin temperature, muscle tension, or even galvanic skin response (a marker of stress), wearables can capture data that offers insights into a person's pain experience.

What's fascinating is that many of these devices go beyond simply tracking one's physical responses. They can also monitor sleep patterns, stress levels, and physical activity—all of which can have a profound impact on pain perception. As chronic pain often involves not just the body but also mental and emotional stress, having access to this data provides us with a more comprehensive understanding of how pain is being experienced.

For example, a wearable device may track when your pain tends to worsen, how it correlates with periods of increased stress, or whether your sleep quality impacts your pain levels. All of this information, when analyzed, can provide us with patterns that can be used to refine your treatment plan.

The Benefits for Patients and Providers

The greatest benefit of wearable technology is that it empowers both patients and healthcare providers. For patients, the ability to track pain levels continuously—without needing to remember every flare-up or write it down in a journal—provides a more accurate reflection of their experience. This real-time data collection can be immensely helpful in discussions with your doctor. It gives us concrete evidence to review during consultations, which can help fine-tune your treatment plan.

As a doctor, I've found that when patients come prepared with detailed data from their wearables, our conversations are much more productive. Instead of relying on general descriptions of pain ("It's been bad this week"), we have precise data that helps identify trends and make more informed decisions. This also allows for more proactive care—if we can see a spike in pain levels or a decline in sleep quality, we can adjust treatment before things escalate into a crisis.

Moreover, many wearables are now equipped with features that alert patients and healthcare providers when certain thresholds are reached, such as when pain increases dramatically or when physical activity levels drop below a certain point. These alerts can act as early warnings, prompting adjustments in therapy, lifestyle changes, or even interventions before things become unmanageable.

The Future of Wearable Pain Monitoring

Looking ahead, the future of wearable technology in chronic pain management is incredibly promising. Devices are becoming increasingly sophisticated, with the potential for even more granular data. Cutting-edge wearables monitor not only physical markers but also emotional states. These technologies are capable of detecting fluctuations in mood and stress levels, which can directly impact pain. Imagine a device that could not only alert you to rising pain levels but also remind you to practice a stress-relieving technique, like deep breathing or meditation, before things get worse.

Wearable tech is also now connecting to other medical devices, like transcutaneous electrical nerve stimulation (TENS) units or even biofeedback systems, so patients can manage their pain in real time. This means that patients could potentially receive treatment on demand—based on the data their wearables provide—giving them more control over their pain.

Challenges and Considerationsconsiderations

Undoubtedly, wearable technology is revolutionizing pain management, yet it still faces challenges that require attention. One of the primary concerns is ensuring the accuracy and reliability of the data collected. While some devices offer highly accurate readings, others may be prone to errors or inconsistencies. Collaborate with your healthcare provider to select an accurate device that meets your requirements.

Another consideration is the accessibility and cost of these devices. While the price of wearables has decreased significantly over the years, they can still represent an additional expense that some patients may not be able to afford. However, as these devices become more mainstream, I believe we will see wider availability and better insurance coverage options.

Integrating Wearables into Pain Management Plans

As your healthcare provider, I see wearables as a complementary tool in a broader, holistic approach to pain management. While they are powerful devices for tracking and monitoring pain, they are not a standalone solution. The best results come when these devices are integrated into a comprehensive pain management plan that includes medical treatment, physical therapy, lifestyle changes, and emotional support.

It's important to remember that wearables cannot replace the expertise and judgment of a skilled healthcare provider. However, they can be an invaluable tool to enhance communication, improve monitoring, and provide real-time data to optimize treatment plans.

In Conclusion

Wearable technology is transforming the way we understand and manage chronic pain. It provides us with real-time, accurate data that empowers both patients and healthcare providers to make better decisions. As a doctor, I've seen how these devices are enhancing our ability to monitor pain, improve treatment outcomes, and provide more personalized care. Despite the challenges ahead, wearable technology in pain management holds promise for more effective and customized solutions.

9.2 Combining Traditional and Modern Practices

As a physician, I have always believed that the most effective approach to pain management is one that embraces the strengths of both traditional and modern practices. Pain is a deeply personal experience, and no single treatment method works for everyone. Whether it's a chronic condition or an acute injury, patients deserve a treatment plan that draws on the best that both modern medicine and traditional healing practices have to offer. Integrating these approaches has revolutionized my practice, yielding numerous benefits for countless patients

The Strengths of Traditional Practices

Traditional medicine, which includes centuries-old practices like acupuncture, Ayurveda, and herbal therapies, has a wealth of knowledge that modern medicine can draw upon. These approaches often focus on treating the root causes of pain, not just the symptoms. For example, acupuncture, which has been practiced for thousands of years, aims to stimulate specific points on the body to release blockages and restore energy flow, helping to reduce pain and inflammation. Similarly, Ayurveda focuses on balancing the body's energies through natural remedies, diet, and lifestyle changes, offering a holistic approach to pain management.

What I have found most compelling about traditional practices is their emphasis on the whole person—body, mind, and spirit. Unlike conventional medicine, which can sometimes be overly focused on diagnosing and treating a specific ailment, traditional practices often approach health from a broader perspective, recognizing the interconnectedness of all aspects of well-being. For patients who feel that modern medicine has only offered them temporary relief or no solution at all, traditional practices can offer a sense of empowerment and self-healing.

The Role of Modern Medicine

On the other hand, modern medicine brings invaluable scientific advances that allow us to diagnose and treat pain with precision and effectiveness. Thanks to cutting-edge imaging technologies, medical procedures, and pharmaceutical innovations, we can address the underlying causes of pain with unprecedented accuracy. From minimally invasive surgeries to biologic treatments like stem cell therapy, modern medicine offers solutions that were once thought impossible.

What's particularly powerful about modern medicine is its ability to intervene in cases where traditional practices alone might not provide sufficient relief. For instance, in cases of acute injury or surgery-related pain, prescription pain medications, nerve blocks, or surgical interventions can offer immediate relief. Furthermore, modern research continues to advance our understanding of pain at the molecular and neurological levels, which gives us a clearer picture of how to treat it effectively.

The Synergy Between Traditional and Modern Approaches

In my experience, the real magic occurs when we integrate traditional and modern practices into a comprehensive treatment plan. I have observed patients experiencing chronic pain, stemming from conditions such as arthritis, fibromyalgia, or others, reap the benefits of a comprehensive approach that integrates the best practices from both fields.

For example, a patient suffering from osteoarthritis may receive pain relief through medication or a joint injection, both of which are modern treatments. However, they might also find significant relief through acupuncture sessions, which can reduce inflammation and improve circulation. Likewise, a patient undergoing physical therapy may supplement their treatment with Ayurvedic herbs or yoga practices to help with flexibility, muscle strength, and stress management. Combining these approaches often leads to better outcomes than either practice alone.

Personalizing the Approach

One of the key aspects of combining traditional and modern practices is personalization. As a physician, it's crucial to understand each patient's unique experience with pain and tailor their treatment accordingly. What works for one patient may not work for another, and that's where a combination of methods can offer a more individualized and adaptive approach.

When I create treatment plans for my patients, I always consider a combination of factors: the nature of their pain, their medical history, their lifestyle, and their preferences. Some patients may be more comfortable with traditional treatments, while others may prefer the latest advancements in medicine. My job is to guide them toward the approach that will offer the best results for them. Not choosing one over the other, but integrating their strengths based on the patient's needs.

Overcoming Challenges

Combining traditional and modern practices can come with its challenges. One of the primary barriers is the lack of understanding or skepticism about the efficacy of traditional treatments in the medical community. Some practitioners may feel that traditional practices are too vague or lack scientific backing. However, as I've seen in my own practice, many traditional approaches are now being validated through modern research, and we are beginning to see how these ancient therapies can complement modern treatments.

There can also be logistical challenges, such as coordinating between multiple healthcare providers—each with different areas of expertise. It requires careful communication and collaboration among physicians, acupuncturists, massage therapists, nutritionists, and other specialists to ensure a cohesive treatment plan. But when the patient is at the center of this collaboration, the benefits far outweigh the difficulties.

A Holistic Approach for the Future

Looking ahead, I believe that the future of pain management lies in a more integrated, holistic approach. Medicine is moving toward a model that combines technology, scientific knowledge, and human-centered care. I see a future where patients have the opportunity to choose from a broad spectrum of treatment options, guided by both their personal preferences and the best available evidence. This approach will empower patients to take charge of their pain journey, supported by a diverse team of healthcare professionals.

Ultimately, pain management is not just about eliminating discomfort. It's about helping patients regain control over their lives, restore function, and enhance their overall well-being. By combining traditional and modern practices, we offer patients a more comprehensive and personalized approach to healing.

In my practice, I am committed to continuing this journey of integration and collaboration. Pain is complex, and the solutions are just as diverse. But with the right combination of old and new, I am confident that we can create a future where pain no longer has to be an unmanageable force in our lives.

Chapter - 10

The Journey

10.1 Remarkable Patient StoriesStories : Lessons from the Frontlines

In my years of practice, I've seen countless individuals battle chronic pain, each facing unique struggles. What stands out to me is not the pain itself, but the strength, determination, and resilience these patients exhibit in the face of immense challenges. Chronic pain is an invisible force that can dictate the course of a person's life, but I've learned that it's not the pain that defines someone—it's their response to it.

What I've come to realize through these years of interaction is that pain is multifaceted. It's not just a physical sensation; it's psychological, emotional, and social. The ways people cope with pain are just as diverse. Some find hope in medical interventions, while others embrace lifestyle changes or a holistic approach to treatment. No matter the path, the underlying theme is that individuals don't just suffer in silence; they fight back, each in their own way.

One of the greatest lessons I've learned from patients is the importance of resilience. While their circumstances may vary, one thing remains constant: the determination to regain control of their lives. Chronic pain can feel like an insurmountable obstacle, but those who rise above it do so by rethinking their relationship with pain and actively seeking solutions. They understand that while pain management isn't an immediate fix, it is a process—one that requires perseverance and collaboration.

Additionally, these experiences have shown me the value of a personalized approach. Each individual's experience with pain is unique, necessitating customized treatments. Some find relief through medication, others through physical therapy, and still others through a combination of alternative therapies. The key takeaway here is that pain is a deeply individual experience, and effective management must take into account not just the pain itself, itself but also the unique circumstances of the person enduring it.

Lastly, the power of self-advocacy unites all these patients. Those who are actively involved in their treatment decisions, who ask questions and seek out the right information, tend to fare better. They don't just accept their diagnosis—they demand a path forward. This kind of empowerment is crucial in the healing process.

In reflecting on the lessons from patients, I've come to appreciate the value of empathy, collaboration, and patience in the treatment of chronic pain. It's a journey for both the patient and the physician. By embracing a holistic approach, a willingness to adapt, and a commitment to empowering patients, we can transform pain management into a more meaningful and effective process.

10.2 A Message of Strength and Hope

To all those living with chronic pain, I want to begin by acknowledging your journey. Pain, especially the kind that lingers and becomes part of your everyday reality, can feel isolating, overwhelming, and, at times, unrelenting. Yet, in my years of working with patients, I've witnessed a remarkable truth: strength is often born out of adversity.

It's straightforward to feel defeated by pain. To believe that your life is limited by what you feel in your body. However, the people I've treated have taught me that pain doesn't define who you are or what you can achieve. Every day, I see individuals who refuse to be defined by their pain, who continue to push forward, who adapt, who rebuild, and who thrive despite the challenges.

Pain may make you feel broken at times, but I urge you to remember that resilience is not about avoiding pain—it's about learning to live alongside it. It's about finding your balance, creating new patterns, and accepting that healing is a process, not an overnight fix. And along the way, there will be setbacks. But it is in those moments of challenge that your inner strength will shine through.

Hope is not a distant concept, reserved only for the end of the journey. You can find hope every day, in small victories, in new insights, and in the decision to keep moving forward. Even when you don't feel like you're making progress—even when the pain seems to dominate—know that your effort matters. Every step you take—no matter how small—is a victory. The journey is not linear, and that's okay. What matters is that you keep moving, keep seeking, and keep hoping.

You are not alone. There is a community of people—doctors, specialists, and patients—who are walking this path with you. We are constantly learning and growing together, and there are solutions out there. It might take time, but there is always hope for relief. It may not look the way you imagined, and the path may not be straightforward, but relief is possible.

I want you to hold onto that hope, and I want you to believe in your strength. The fight against chronic pain is one of endurance, but you are more than capable of navigating it. You have already demonstrated immense courage by seeking help, continuing to explore options, and refusing to accept that pain marks the end of your story.

So, take heart. Pain does not define you. Your ability to rise above it, to live your life with purpose, and to keep going despite the obstacles is the true measure of your strength. Continue to focus on the future, maintain faith in the potential for better days, and never forget that healing—mental, emotional, and physical—is a journey worth embarking on. You are stronger than you think, and there is always hope.